KATE GROSS was thirty-six years old when she died from colon cancer at her home in Cambridge on Christmas morning 2014. Before her cancer, Kate read English at Oxford University. She joined the civil service and worked in Number 10 Downing Street for Tony Blair and Gordon Brown. On leaving, she worked with Tony Blair to found the Africa Governance Initiative, a charity which works to rebuild structures of government in post-conflict Africa. She was awarded an OBE in 2014 for her work. She began to write a blog after her initial diagnosis which can be found at kateelizabethgross.word-press.com. She is survived by her husband Billy and their five-year-old sons Isaac and Oscar.

From the reviews of *Late Fragments*:

'Boy, does [Kate's] writing have pulse. Clear-sighted and cold-eyed, her sentences are light as leaves and she was as wise as a magi … When [her twins] wonder about their mother, here she will be, bold and brave, caught on the page in all her wonderful vitality'

FRANCIS WILSON, *Mail on Sunday*, 5*

'Raw, honest, yet unexpectedly positive … A warm and oddly uplifting read. Gross is funny in the darkest moments of truth. Neither falsely upbeat nor purpose-fully dramatic or tear-jerking, the book brings Gross to life, and she feels to the reader like a friend, or at least someone you would like to have known'

RACHAEL PELLS, *Independent*

'Life lessons that only someone staring death in the face could impart ... With her lucid prose and piercing perception Kate is as much of a loss to the world of literature as she is to politics ... Her determined positivity breaks through time and again ... How can you fail to admire such strength in the face of adversity? ... She tells her story with unflinching honesty. You just wish its ending were different'

CHARLOTTE HEATHCOTE, *Daily Express*, 5*

'Gross is an elegant and straightforward writer, sprinkling wit and bitterness in all the right places. She strikes a balance between putting the reader in her shoes and expressing the impossible solitude of facing what you have to face ... It is extremely difficult to write on this subject evocatively, but without sentimentality ... [Kate] treats herself as a case study, a bystander with a story to tell. The effect is readable, engaging and enriching ... To do that as your final act is amazing'

VIV GROSKOP, *Daily Telegraph*, 5*

'It is overwhelmingly sad, but it's not maudlin or self-pitying. Instead, there is a sense of wonder, a determination to live and love with her whole heart in the little time she has left ... Funny and sharp and celebratory'

SARAH FRANKLIN, *Sunday Express*, 5*

'This brave, lucid, witty memoir succeeds in expressing the essence of Kate to people who will only ever know her through its pages' *Daily Mail*

'She moves us into the sun with her. Her tone is witty, always serious, but rarely solemn. Her prose is grounded, unshowy and blessed with a casual poetry ... To read this book is to learn what can be snatched back from death ... her attitude is worth the sky'

ROBERT WEBB, *New Statesman*

'Gross writes with steadfast, exquisite skill and although this remarkable book is hard to get through without a box of hankies, it is also one of the most galvanising you are likely to read all year. She wanted to pass on the gift of wonder to her sons; her gift to her reader is to inspire them to live life with as much joy, hunger and gusto as she did – READ IT AND LEAP'

CLAIRE ALLFREE, *Metro*

'She didn't always know she was going to die young. But she lived as if she might. In other words, there was no wastage in Kate's life ... *Late Fragments* is a gem – a wonderful, uplifting reflection on how to die and how to live ... There is nothing tragic about its message which is a happy one, full of life's possibilities, not its limitations. The lesson is that it is not the longevity of your life but the intensity of it which counts; that what you give lasts longer than what you take; and that if you contribute, even to the smallest degree, to the betterment of human-kind then you will not be a memory but a living and moving spirit that even after death can change the world around you. Such a spirit is Kate'

TONY BLAIR, *Sunday Times*

'*Late Fragments* is so beautiful'   HADLEY FREEMAN

'Gross was that rare mix, of intellect and empathy… The book's power lies in the unflinching way she shares her life's lessons and how she rationalises what it's really like to be told "you are going to die" … It's like getting a crash course on the meaning of life through the medium of literature … Her thoughts on friendship, family, love and loss preoccupied me for days, pulling me back through the book to read through certain passages again and again … Hers is a voice that is clear and spirited from a woman who was funny, clever and wise'

JACKIE ANNESLEY, *Sunday Times*

'As [Kate's] extraordinarily frank, funny and heart-breaking book shows, the cancer couldn't take away that "kernel of Kate" she describes so brilliantly within its pages … *Late Fragments* tells of a life truly lived'

Vanity Fair

'Gross herself seems not to have been floored by her early death sentence … Separating the darks from the lights is one of her own great talents. Among the many things to appreciate in Gross's honest, intelligent and deeply affect-ing book is her observation that the intensity of terminal illness makes it perversely animating, that only death, in other words, can make the most out of life'

CLAIRE HARMAN, *Guardian*

'More than a cancer memoir – it is also a superb manual for living. Highly recommended' MATTHEW D'ANCONA

'[An] uplifting memoir of a life taken too soon … [Kate's] story is equal parts moving and humbling'
PAUL FLYNN, *Grazia*

'Heart-stopping, hankie-soaking, true, sad and funny … A book that, in every page, lives and breathes the wise old lesson we often learn too late – that dying teaches us how to live. It does that not with soulful platitudes, but with blunt honesty laced with a wicked sense of humour. I imagine, if you knew Kate, that it would sound exactly like her … Kate has left a gift for anyone who chooses to pick up this book. It is the gift of wonder, if only we can find it, and the reminder that no matter what happens to you, "you are the captain of your soul". It's you that gets to choose how you react to whatever happens to you in life. So, first, read her wise words. Then go give your life meaning – your way' LAUREN HADDEN, *Psychologies*

'[Kate has] that power to see just that little bit further than most people, to bring clarity to an idea or to a conversation that for most other people had begun to blur on the boundaries of their horizon … *Late Fragments* is not merely about living and dying at far too young an age. It is about the joy of family and friends, of falling in love' TOM PECK, *Independent*

'[A] wise, luminous book ... it will mean a great deal to a lot of people ... Gross has written a book that is full of joy, and I finished vowing to live as much and as hard as I can'   SAMANTHA ELLIS, *Literary Review*

'Very powerful writing ... Immediate, fearless, often blackly funny ... Gross is a gifted writer, with an innate sense of the right words in the right order. It is impossible to read her without being pulled up short: inspired by her joy in life, thankful for your own health, moved that this family is still functioning, wondering what you would do in the same situation ... A memoir about both how to die and how to live, it is funny and wise ... The book is a remarkable final achievement for a woman who cares about putting something back – even when everything is being taken away'   LOUISE FRANCE, *The Times*

'*Late Fragments* is something of a masterpiece. Powerful and painfully honest, Kate writes lyrically and effortlessly about family, growing up, love, friendship, her passion for literature – and about the importance of finding wonder in everyday life'
EMMA HIGGINBOTHAM, *Cambridge News*

Kate Gross

Late Fragments

Everything I Want to Tell You
(About this Magnificent Life)

**WILLIAM
COLLINS**

William Collins
An imprint of HarperCollins*Publishers*
1 London Bridge Street
London SE1 9GF

First published by William Collins in 2014
This William Collins paperback edition published 2015
1

Permission to quote from 'Black Rook in Rainy Weather' by Sylvia Plath has been kindly
granted by Faber and Faber Ltd. 'Late Fragments' and 'What the Doctor Said', from
All Of Us: Collected Poems by Raymond Carver (Harvill Secker), copyright © Tess
Gallagher, 1996, used by permission of The Wylie Agency (UK) Limited and the Random
House Group Ltd. Grateful acknowledgement is made to The Wylie Agency for electronic
rights to quote material from Raymond Carver. Permission to quote from Rohinton
Mistry's *Family Matters* also kindly granted by Faber and Faber Ltd. Lyrics from 'The Joy
of Living' by Ewan MacColl reprinted with kind permission of Ewan MacColl Ltd.
Thanks to Becs Andrews and Nadia Bettega for the illustrations.

A catalogue record for this book is
available from the British Library

ISBN 978-0-00-810347-7

Printed and bound in Great Britain by
Clays Ltd, St Ives plc

MIX
Paper from
responsible sources
FSC® C007454

There are two copies of this book that matter. There are two pairs of eyes I imagine reading every word. There are two adult hands which I hope will hold a battered paperback when others have long forgotten me and what I have to say. I write this for Oscar and Isaac, my little Knights, my joy and my wonder.

Contents

Introduction

When I was three, I told my mum that I kept my words in my head, in a clear plastic bag. Now it is time for me to take them out, to arrange them into this story. The thing is, I don't know how it ends. I don't know if I will die before I finish writing it. But if I do, I know someone else will write the ending for me. My mum will step in to close off my story, just as she used to step in to help with my homework. So I can begin.

We will start on 11 October 2012. I am running along the beach in Southern California. It is dusk, and as the waves break on the shore, surfers head out to sea. My legs feel strong, my lungs full of salty air. I'm here to raise money for the charity I run, which works in post-conflict Africa. I'm a successful thirty-something woman with an amazing job through which I travel the world and converse with presidents and prime ministers. My adorable twins are three, and their father, Billy, is my soulmate, as well as being the best-looking man I've ever kissed. But inside me a lump of cells has broken free of the rules and spawned a tumour which has blocked my colon, crept through my lymph nodes and colonised my liver. Cancer is halfway to killing me, and I am completely oblivious to its presence.

The next day I am at the airport, my week-long trip over, and finally on my way home to Cambridge. As I arrive at check-in, I am hit by a wave of nausea. I throw up for fifteen hours – through security, in the lounge, and all the way back home. I feel feverish, exhausted. Now, at last, I know something is seriously wrong. I crawl into a taxi at Heathrow and ask the driver to drop me off at the emergency department at Addenbrooke's, our local hospital. A CT scan follows, and twelve hours after landing in the UK I am in emergency surgery. The blockage in my colon is a tumour, and the dark spots the doctors saw on my liver a series of secondary lesions – metastases, to use the proper term. I have stage four cancer. All this cancer-speak is new to me, but I do know there isn't a stage five. What I didn't realise then – though of course the ever internet-enabled Billy did, right from the start – was that I had only a 6 per cent chance of surviving the next five years.

Now we are more than two years on from that, the first earthquake to hit our little family. Two operations, six months of chemotherapy, and a brief, joyful remission filled that interlude. But now the cancer is back. It has spread, it is incurable. I will die before my children finish primary school, and probably before they reach the grand old age of six, which they think is impossibly grown-up, and I think is impossibly young. It won't be long now.

I began to write straight after my diagnosis. And as soon as I started to type, the words emerged, as prolific at reproducing and ordering themselves as the malignant cells inside me. Everything I wrote was a gift to myself, a reminder that I could create even as my body tried to self-destruct. And I wrote as a gift to those I love: my living, breathing Terracotta Army. Now the words spill out of my plastic bag like the magnetic letters my children stick on the fridge. I write to make sense of what has happened to our family, to make sense of the Kate who has emerged in this strange, lucid final chunk of life. I write because the imprint of disease is growing in me, and like a poor man's Keats I find myself full of fears that I will have to stop 'before my pen has glean'd my teeming brain'. Before I can write down all the things I want to tell my boys when they are thirty-five, not five. Before I can tell them who I am, and what I know, and the stories that make up my life.

Someone asked me what was the best thing cancer had given me. I collapsed inside when she said that. Cancer is a pretty terrible kind of gift. It takes and takes and takes, leaving a trail of destruction in its path. It's taken the future I had planned for myself: a career doing Good Things, travelling the world, being important and successful on the terms I had long set myself. It's stolen the take-it-for-granted ease from my relationship with Billy. What's easy about being thirty-six and having your husband nurse you in your dying days? We should be bickering about who takes the bins out, not having heart-to-hearts about how I want our children raised. It's taken away my ability to care for others – by now, I should be helping out my parents, but instead they are visiting me in hospital and picking my kids up from school. They are suddenly 'spare' parents, not grandparents. It's taken the reciprocity out of relationships. Suddenly I am the visited, never the visitor; the receiver, not the sender of cards and presents. And it's taken away my ability to be the mother I want to be. Where I should be careless, bossy, energetic and distracted, now I am diligent, soft and weak, because I can't bear to be remembered as bad cop. Every cuddle is charged with electric joy at their being *there*, and misery that I won't see their future. I find myself lying in their beds as they sleep, crying hot tears into their pudgy necks.

But disease gives as well as it takes. Or, more accurately, we take from it even in the face of its efforts to take everything from us. And so my friend was sort-of-right. What disease has stolen is the normality I took for granted and the future I would have had. But I have taken from it, too. For starters, there is a feeling of being alive, awake, which power-fully reasserts itself in the moments of wellness that punctuate a long illness. I can only explain this feel-ing as rather like your first time on Ecstasy, but with less pounding music and projectile vomiting. Whether it is emerging from chemotherapy, or waking up after operations, I have experienced joy – perhaps even the sublime – in an unexpected and new way. The first time this happened was in the incongruous setting of Ward L4, on the night after my first diagnosis. I opened a window in the middle of the night and leaned out to feel the cold autumn rain on my face, mingling with sharp, blissed-out tears.

Then there is the way I feel about the people in my life. Billy and I have grown a love known only in power ballads, a depth of understanding and companionship which in any fair world would last us a lifetime. My parents, now closer physically as well as emotionally. Friendships which survived on the leftover bits of time have had a renaissance. And while I like to imagine that the world may have lost a future stateswoman, I have found my voice, and with my voice an intellectual and spiritual hinterland which had been lost for too long between the answering of emails and the wiping of tiny bottoms. I am woman, hear me roar.

So despite all that has been and will be taken from us, I am happy. I am really, truly happy. These last years have been so strangely luminous, full of exploration, wonder and love. I'm not sure if this adds up to a silver lining, whether it amounts to enough to balance the loss of the future I should have had. Some days it seems crazy even to suggest it. But it at least makes the scales more even.

I am writing this book to share the sum of a life. In a normal world, I would have been granted decades to say all of this. Fat, old and wearing purple, I would have bored my children and my children's children with stories of the world I had known. Perhaps they would have asked me about the crazy Noughties, the dying days of capitalism, what it was like working in the heart of government when America was king and credit was easy. Or perhaps they would have been more interested in my stories about Africa in the bad old days of hunger and warlords, before Lagos became a place you emigrated to, not from. Maybe they would just have wanted to know what my favourite books were as a child, what my earliest memories were, about how Billy and I fell in love. But I am living at an accelerated pace now. We won't have those conversations; but my children will always have these words.

1

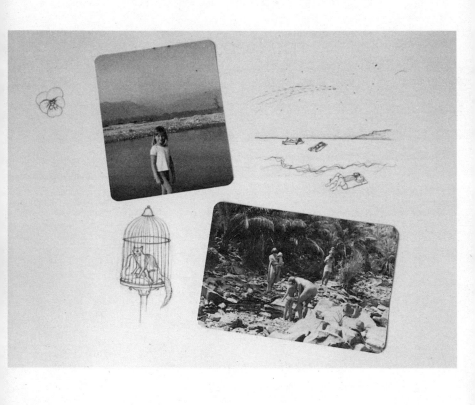

The Plastic Bag and
the Red Coat

A certain minor light may still
Leap incandescent

Out of kitchen table or chair
As if a celestial burning took
Possession of the most obtuse objects now and
    then –
Thus hallowing an interval
Otherwise inconsequent

By bestowing largesse, honour,
One might say love.

SYLVIA PLATH, 'BLACK ROOK IN RAINY WEATHER'

There was a moment, a decade or so ago, when I was walking across Clapham Common on a grey winter day. The sky was flat and far too close to my head. I was in a no-particular-sort-of-mood, probably on my way to spending an afternoon in the pub. Or shopping. Anyway: engaging in delightful, consumerist, meaningless modern life. And then I saw a child in a red coat, and I experienced a moment of absolute, pure wonder. Joy, transcendent and uplifting. Did I borrow this memory from the film *Schindler's List*? Or perhaps this unexpected moment of joy reminded me of watching a scene from another film, *American Beauty*, in which the teenage antihero films a plastic bag with tender attention as it swirls around, suspended in the air, capturing every twist and flutter. No, I believe this memory is my own: there is wonder in the everyday, if you can only see it.

I am not pretending that I go round all the time having this kind of experience. Or that I see it only in red coats, or indeed in plastic bags. It is just that if I could give my children one thing, it would be this capacity to be astonished by the quotidian, to experience joy from the world they live in. I would work out its formula and put it into a pair of super-hero glasses – me and the former dean of Westminster Michael Mayne both, who wrote in his letters to his grandchildren: 'If I could have waved a fairy wand at your birth and wished upon you just one gift it would not have been beauty or riches or a long life: it would have been the gift of wonder.' But it doesn't work like that. We all have to find wonder for ourselves. All I can do is explain how wonder emerged for me as the world and I met, and how it has grown stronger and brighter even as my world has got smaller and dimmer.

I can spread my childhood memories out like a patchwork quilt. My quilt is brightly coloured, richly textured, a mix of the familiar and the foreign. My parents showed me the world from an early age, and experiencing it – drinking in the astonishing wonder it provides – has made me who I am. Because of them, 'the ears of my ears awake and the eyes of my eyes are open', as ee cummings put it. Aged about four, I saw a mongoose eat a snake on the banks of the Creek in Dubai. We used to go into the city on a Friday night for curry. In one corner of the garden of the small and scruffy café by the water sat a big cage. And inside the cage lived a mongoose, and the mongoose was fed snakes. After our curry we would have freshly squeezed fruit juice in a small bar staffed by nice Indian men who would pinch my fat, freckly Caucasian cheeks. I remember our weekend trips to the beach, where we would camp under enormous, starry skies. In 1986, age seven and three quarters, I lay on the cold sand with my friend Georgia, and watched Halley's Comet fly overhead. We made a solemn promise that we would watch it together on its next cycle through the sky, when Georgia will be in her eighties and I will be long gone. During the hot, cloudless days we would blow up our inflatable lilos and drift out into the clear waters of the Persian Gulf in search of the Utter East. In the shallow seas, stingrays lurked under the rocks along with the cuttlefish. At night we children would whisper ghost stories in our tents as the heat of the day gave way to the cold desert night, until we were lulled to sleep by the sounds of our parents drinking cold beers around the campfire.

Because I was brought up far away, in a dusty, dry place where the inside of our blue Toyota was like a metal furnace most of the year round, England felt very foreign to me. Our summers spent in the Wiltshire countryside were as full of wonder as anything I experienced abroad – the everyday stuff of an English childhood rendered foreign by the exotica of my life on the Arabian Peninsula. I remember sunshine and an abundance of soft grass, so different from the scratchy Astroturf of our garden in Dubai. Smooth green banks of grass to roll down, to somersault over, to play leapfrog on. Delicate, pastel-coloured flowers waiting for me to snip them and stuff them in my flower press; flowers which for the first time in my experience looked as if they might actually house fairies, unlike the gargantuan, ferocious flora of the Middle East. Gentle, small butterflies landing on the buddleia outside Court House in our little village of Bishopstone, waiting for me to swoop in with my net. Paddling in too-cold streams with trousers rolled up, learning how to build dams.

As a family, we are travellers. Exploring is part of our DNA, just as much as being shortsighted. We are addicted to the smell of *elsewhere* which hits when you descend from a plane, the excitement of buying milk in a foreign supermarket. My grandfather spent his war in the intelligence corps, in India and Burma, and returned to India with the BBC afterwards. Mum remembers the presents he brought home: exotic silks and carvings, and stories of a place which captivated him. In Kathmandu, when I was six, I saw the Living Goddess, a girl about my age who was locked inside an ornately carved wooden house, with dark kohled eyes and a shiny red and gold dress. How I envied her then, being chosen to be a goddess. But I thought she looked so sad, and as though she wanted very much to be able to play as I could. In Thailand I smelled the cloying odour of durian fruit while we floated down the khlongs of Bangkok. Butterflies of incredible size and colour flitted around me as we walked through the jungle. Black leeches attached themselves to our feet and legs as we hopped over enormous puddles and overflowing rivers in the pouring rain. As a child brought up in the desert, this was my first encounter with the many-shaded green of the tropics, the clichéd wonder of independent travel which would only grow during my university holidays.

There are so many places I wanted to take my boys. Places I have been and seen, and places I have not. To India, to see the coracles floating down the river at Hampi and to hear stories of the oldest civilisations. To Vietnam, to eat soft-shell crabs on a street corner while you watch the future take shape in the concrete flyovers and skyscrapers above you. To California, to experience everything super-sized, including the boundless optimism and confidence of the glossy-haired, honey-limbed natives. To Africa, to see the misty thousand hills in Rwanda and to understand how a people can tear themselves apart and remake themselves in a generation, because history is not a death sentence. To Egypt, or maybe Morocco, to see souks and pyramids, riads and the simple, mesmerising shapes of Islamic art. To mountain ranges where you feel the bliss of solitude as you glide in a silent chairlift amidst deep, silent snowdrifts. To tropical seas as clear as glass, where you can enter another world underwater, watching turtles and stingrays glide through shoals of magically coloured fish.

I won't take my children to those places now. But still, I try to guess how and where they will experience the wonder that will make them see the world anew. Perhaps it has already come, in the Botanic Garden in Cambridge. There, we run round the lake, climb mountains, explore jungles and cross rivers on stepping stones, and are still only a mile from our front door. Or in the places we have already been: stretching our legs to cross the slippery stones of the Giant's Causeway, with the myths of Finn McCool ringing in our ears. Or in the magical house in France my dad built, where it never rains, the swimming pool is always blue, and a snake called Oliver Cromwell lives under the veranda.

The point is, I don't know how they will experience the world, any more than I can guide them through it. I hope that its breadth and variety will provide them with the endless thrill it has for me. But staying at home is fine too. I need them to know that wonder doesn't require a passport, it only requires your attention. My dad has always been evidence of that. He's a traveller too, and he told me once about wonder emerging for him as he surveyed the wild cliffs of St David's in Wales as a long-haired, dope-smoking student (remember, it was the Seventies). But his truest sense of wonder has always been found in a smaller world around him. He sees things, you see, in the details: the curve of a white tulip petal, the way a tree branch stretches over a lake, the perfect structure of the green hills and the flat causse near the house he built in France. Like Emily Dickinson, his holy trinity is the Bee, the Butterfly and the Breeze. He is a man who takes joy from his surroundings, someone who like Thomas Hardy considers himself a man who *notices* things.

How strange, how brilliant it is that this awareness of wonder, this sense of the sublime, has been so closely intertwined with my illness as it has progressed. How incredible that Ruskin's duty to delight in the world around has grown stronger in me as I have grown weaker.

But before I go any further, I had better tell the story of how the cancer inside me – the beast I know as the Nuisance – started, because it is the frame for everything else that follows.

I've always had a dodgy bottom. I presumed it was irritable bowel syndrome. I guessed it had been exacerbated by the various terrible afflictions of the innards I obtained while working in India, where I taught for a few months post-university. Within a month of arriving there I was sustaining myself only by gulab jamun, the gelatinous, sticky Indian sweets. Everything else on the school's menu, including the inoffensive-seeming parathas, had left me squatting painfully over the stand-up loos or running out of assembly to vomit in the verdant flowerbeds. Clearly, I thought, there was some mutant worm growing inside me. I nuked it with antibiotics when I got home, but I seemed to be left with something permanently wrong down there. In a very British style, I ignored it valiantly for about seven years. By then, I was anyway busy with being a young and ambitious worker bee, and falling in love.

It was only when I paused and left London that I vowed to get my health sorted out. We had moved to Cambridge – home of Billy's technology start-up, which he'd founded the very month he and I went on our first date, in 2004. It was my turn to do the commute to London, but I was avoiding that, and indeed reality in general, by going back to university to do a Masters. Being a student again gave me plenty of time to go and get things checked out. After I had described my symptoms to my GP, she sent me off to hospital, where they put a little camera up my bottom. The nice consultant found nothing to worry about, and told me to eat more fibre to regularise things down there. Little did I know, not being the bottom-health expert I now am, that I had only had a sigmoidoscopy: in layman's terms, a camera that peeks only partway up your arse, rather than exploring the whole lot. If the camera had poked a bit further round my innards, the consultant probably would have found an adenoma, a pre-cancerous little polyp in my colon. He would have cut it out, I would have been booked in for regular screening, and life would have proceeded to plan. But that didn't happen. To make matters worse, I always confidently told subsequent doctors I had had a clear colonoscopy, and that everything down there was Just Fine.

In any case, the ensuing years were eventful for other, more pressing reasons. With (I thought) my health problems sorted, I got pregnant in 2008. My twelve-week scan revealed two little swimmers thrashing around in my uterus. Twin boys. Billy and I were petrified. Like cancer, twins didn't run in the family. What were the chances? One in eighty, apparently, significantly greater than the one in twenty thousand chance of getting colon cancer aged thirty-four. But back to the story. In May 2009 my little swimmers emerged, full-term and healthy. Motherhood took over my body and my mind, as is its way. I was swept along on a wave of oxytocin, and apart from the sleep deprivation felt happier and healthier than I ever had.

Being a mother consumed me, and what energy was left over I applied to work. Halfway through my Masters I had set up the Africa Governance Initiative, working again for our former prime minister Tony Blair. Not only was he the smartest, kindest and most relaxed politician I had ever worked for, he also had a belief in the role of government as a force for good which profoundly appealed to my public-servant heart. He wanted to use what he'd learned in ten long years in power for the benefit of some of the poorest people in the world, by working with the leaders of Africa's emerging democracies, countries coming out of years of war and mismanagement. As someone who had always seen myself as a bureaucrat with the heart of an explorer, this seemed like a perfect fit. With Tony working alongside presidents and prime ministers, the charity we founded put teams of international staff – capable, passionate, bright young things – into the heart of burgeoning democracies, countries like Liberia, Rwanda and Sierra Leone. There we worked with many incredible African public servants, sitting alongside them in bombed-out, sweltering buildings, with more chickens in the corridors than staff in the offices, assisting with the task of rebuilding a country and shaping a fair, effective and clean government. Between wrangling with twins and being CEO of this new enterprise, I didn't have much time to worry as my old bottom troubles worsened. Anyway, it was all too easy to blame things on the Rwandan goat brochettes.

Fast forward to October 2012. The kids are three and a bit. I am thirty-four, and something inside just doesn't feel right. I am very, very tired. On Saturdays I stick the boys in front of the TV while I sleep. I go to the GP. I tell her I've had a colonoscopy. She asks when. I say 2007, and she tells me they are valid for five years. Now the problems really begin. I start getting terrible abdominal pains. These reach a peak during an excruciatingly dull interview I'm conducting for a new chief operating officer. Suddenly, it feels as if a giant boulder has rolled across my intestines – a pretty accurate metaphor, it turns out, if you exchange 'boulder' for 'tumour'. But still, life continues. A return trip to the GP, who tells me I probably have a blockage down there, but it's nothing to worry about. I wonder whether, if my problems had been in a less, well, shitty area (say my armpit) I would have fought harder over the years to sort them out.

But I didn't, and so off I go to California, to running on Laguna Beach, to that accursed United Airlines flight home, and to the CT scan and finally the operating table on 12 October when my tumour and its liverish little friends finally come to light.

I woke up after the operation with Billy next to my hospital bed. It was he who told me, then, that I definitely had cancer. He was reassuring, gentle, a little wild-eyed but surprisingly calm. I was euphoric, full of morphine, and overjoyed to see him. Terrified of my first general anaesthetic, I hadn't really expected to wake up from the operation. But there I was, on a general surgery ward, midnight on a Friday, with a diagnosis of advanced cancer. And ecstatic to be alive.

God knows what it had been like for Billy to get my phone calls that day: first, telling him I was in hospital. Next, that I'd had a scan and was likely to need surgery. Then, just an hour later, that there was a chance it might be cancer, and that they were operating immediately. He stayed with me right up until I was wheeled into surgery, then walked away. He told me afterwards that while I was under the knife he sat in our little garden smoking and crying. The surgeon had rung him afterwards and confirmed the worst. Then, in the dead of night, Billy came in to be by my side when I woke up. And as I drifted back off into my euphoric, opiated haze he returned home to scour the internet for survival strategies, treatments and miracle cures.

Gentle reader, you may have the misfortune to know all about cancer already. If so, forgive me for what follows. Cancer comes in four easy-to-remember stages. Picture your body as a house – your 'bone-house', as it was called by the Anglo-Saxon poets – and cancer as your formerly domesticated dog, now running wild and intent on rampaging through the neighbourhood, destroying all in his path. Stage one is 'local' cancer, your dog confined to your kitchen: just the one bodily organ. Here he can make mayhem, but be relatively easily tamed and managed. In stage two, your dog has managed to outgrow the kitchen, and has burst through the wall to colonise the living room, getting his messy hairs and doggy smell everywhere. Taming this beast and removing the traces of him will now be harder.

Stage three sees Dog getting all the way to the front door and bounding out (with the front door being the lymph nodes, in this tortured analogy). You can shut the door at this point, but once the blighter has tasted freedom it's hard to contain his desire to explore the neighbourhood. And so stage four comes. Here, Dog has run amok, taken a giant crap on the pavement, eaten out of the bins and settled into the chippy down the road for a snooze. Your cancer has spread from its initial home to other vital organs. Because of our inability to speak of our rear ends, most colon cancer is detected somewhere between stages two and four, and the chances of cure decline dramatically as the patient progresses through the stages.

But in the hospital that weekend, I don't yet know any of this. Billy researches the statistics for me. Over time he tells me that while my prognosis is poor, the numbers apply to old people, and since I am so young and healthy I am *bound* to have a better shot at things. The information on the internet is about five years out of date, and new treatments, surgical techniques and so on have bumped up survival rates.

If the tumours in my liver can be operated on, I actually have a chance of a complete recovery – admittedly it's still only fifty–fifty, if we even get that far. But those odds feel brilliant to us at this stage.

There were a lot of ifs, in those first few weeks. I could explain them all, and all the ups and downs that followed during the next months of chemotherapy through till my liver operation, and then the reappearance of the Nuisance all over my body six months later. But that would litter the pages of this whole book with jargon, and make it incomprehensibly, boringly medical. It is enough to say that as Billy and I looked ahead in those strange hours after my operation, we saw a landscape of uncertainty. My vision was blurred by morphine and pain. His was sharper, and he could see, more clearly than I, the life we had thought stretched before us disappear into a fog of disease, hospitals, statistics, and just plain luck.

But through the haze I had my first taste of the bitter gratitude that has accompanied my diagnosis. I have already told you about the almost transcendental experience I had feeling the soft October rain on my face as I stumbled from my hospital bed to lean out of the window after the operation, and the joyful feeling of aliveness which consumed my mind and body despite having been told I might die. But there were more practical things that brought me joy too. First, everyone else on my ward had stoma – or colostomy – bags. I never actually saw one, but I knew that they lurked under the baggy hospital gowns, catching the poo from the piece of the colon that peeked out of the stomach, a second bottom carved by surgeons in many, many abdominal operations. Somehow, my genius surgeon had managed to piece me back together without the need for one of those things. Second, though my body had let me down by allowing this cancer to take root, it had also propelled me home. Somehow, it had found the strength to travel five and a half thousand miles back to Cambridge to receive this unreceivable news in the only place I could bear it. And so there I was, the old world around me crashing down. Everything I had taken for granted swept away. And yet I was full to the brim with an irrepressible joy.

* * *

Back to now. No more smell of hot *elsewhere* as I disembark from a plane. Life is quiet. My joy comes from small things; no travel documents required. I watch the crocuses pop up on the Cambridge Backs, little purple and orange heralds of the winter thawing. The bare trees in the park at the end of our road look like an Aubrey Beardsley etching on the big East Anglian sky. I swim in the sea in Devon, too early in the year for those sensible people with time to spare. Breaking the oncologist's rules, I feel the thrill of dangerous, wild nature enfold me as hypothermia rises from my feet upwards. I roll over to Billy in the morning and watch him sleep, nosily at peace. Reading *Four Quartets*, the words imprint my mind, filling me with amazement at how Eliot grapples with the sense of time that haunts me. 'At the still point, there the dance is.' I search for the still point every day, and sometimes I even manage to find some peace there, because, after all, there *is* only the dance.

There is wonder in my past, and in my present. As I write this book, I lay out my memory quilt to see all the dancing I have done: places I have been, people I have met. I have fitted so much colour into my short life that I wonder if I lived on hyper-speed, as if, somehow, I knew my time was limited.

Soon my wonder will come from watching the tree outside my window as it shakes in the sky, and from my children curling their small hands around mine. My world will shrink to one room. But I know wonder will still assail me.

2

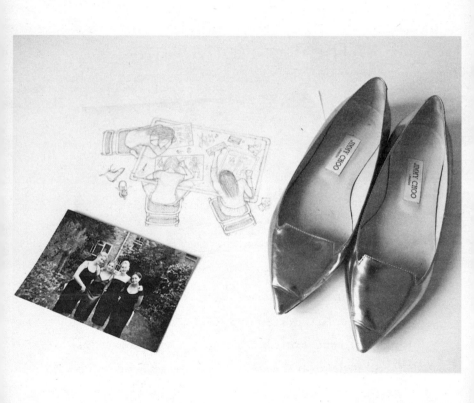

The Terracotta Army

My friends are my 'estate'.

EMILY DICKINSON

Once upon a time there was a girl who lived in a town of hills and honey-coloured stone, where putrid steam rose from ancient hot springs, and it almost always rained. The girl was called Kate, and she was a teenager. Kate was an unpleasant creature, because back then she didn't know who she was. Really, as a foetid little grub she should have been cocooned in a dark chamber for ten years before emerging as a bright, sparkling (stealthily cancer-ridden) butterfly, but a defect in human evolution means this most unpleasant and painful of developmental stages is carried out in the glare of daylight. And it was only when Kate finally hatched out and shed her caterpillar skin that she found the people who have walked with her ever since. The people who have made life like Oz, even when gloom, pain and drugs sucked the Technicolor from the world and tried to turn it to Kansas.

This was originally going to be the chapter which provided a bit of light relief, some laughs to relieve the solemnity of a book about dying. But writing it is, strangely, more painful for me than anything else, because being a teenager – and specifically the years thirteen to sixteen – were without doubt the worst period of my life. Yes, really. Far worse than my acquaintance with the Nuisance. As far as I can tell, becoming who you are as an adult requires a period wherein you are possessed by a wicked spirit who hates everything. Your childhood. Your parents. Old friends. Your bedroom. Your clothes. Your face. It's messy to watch, and even messier on the inside. But it's Darwinian, a necessary stratagem for the self to evolve into something which is no longer a child, and which can survive and thrive outside the nest. So

I shall provide some gruesome details of the grub years, because in every good story there is a period of despair before hope arrives.

Back to Kate, in her blue bedroom in the small, honey-coloured town, nestled amongst seven hills like a damp, Austen-ified version of Rome. I kept a diary. At the start of 1992 it began with the line, 'It is January. But which January?' (This arch opener because I expected my juvenilia to be anthologised one day.) But there wasn't anything dramatic about that January, or indeed any other January at that point in my life. After the holidays I went back to my slightly-better-than-bog-standard comprehensive school. There are two pertinent facts about this school. First, the existence of a wonderful English teacher. Second, it was single-sex. No boys. This gave it a particularly rank smell of female sweat and cruelty, the sort that only gets dished out girl-on-girl. Back then, friendships were toxic, obsessional things. The wound of my first ever best friend Rosie Lee (who I loved for her curly blonde hair and extensive knowledge of Kylie Minogue lyrics) leaving me for another still smarts. One day, I was cast aside on the long walk to school in favour of Katrina. Katrina was older than Rosie and me. Worldly. But Rosie provided no explanation for this abandonment. There was no process of separation, no divorce. I trailed behind them day after day like a sad Labrador, silently ignored.

This was my first realisation that I was not one of the cool girls. It would have been hard to be cool, looking as I did in 1992. First, there was my hair, which was coloured bright orange with henna. My fringe was blunt. I had many freckles and a very round face, and even rounder tortoiseshell glasses. Then, as now, I was quite sturdy ('Built like the rest of us Tanner gals!' my heftily-bosomed grandmother would say brightly). Though my name sounded like hers, I was basically the antithesis of Kate Moss. The fashion, back then, was grunge, which is ideal teen-age wear: grubby, shapeless old clothes, band T-shirts and tie-dye. My favourite outfit that January was a pair of bottle-green corduroy culottes paired with purple tights and one of my hand tie-dyed T-shirts (with Dr Martens boots, of course). Someone else – say, Kate Moss, or my erstwhile friend Rosie Lee –

probably could have rocked this look. But it's safe to say I didn't really own it; I let the corduroy culottes wear me, and that is something no woman should ever write. So neither the way I looked, nor the way I dressed, was particularly beneficial in helping me to join the school Cooliverse I so longed to be part of.

My brain was a problem too. There was something profoundly uncool about being clever, at least at my school. I was one of those children who are desperate to please teachers, who work *very hard* and do *very well*. I got enough As to bump up the school's shonky results, had enough gumption to ask interesting questions in class, but not enough attitude to be disruptive. It didn't help that I had no cool hobbies. I never really got into pop music; books were my thing, which was marginally better than playing the trumpet, but nonetheless not conducive to being kissed. So, as time went on, I started going to ever-greater lengths to hide my nerdish and teacher-pleasing tendencies. I made a show of falling asleep in lessons, so that it looked as if I had the kind of social life I coveted. I skipped physics, because poor old Mr Whale didn't really notice whether we were there or not. I didn't stop getting good results – diligence prevailed, and I pored over my books outside school, where I could indulge my owlish obsessions under the safe wings of the wonderful ladies of literature my mum had wisely chosen as her friends (especially my godmother Louise and my friend's mum Susie, both English teachers). But at school, I stopped being an interested, engaged student. I stopped being proud of what went on in my head. And worst of all, like Rosie Lee, I cast aside the friendships I had with people who talked to me about books in favour of people who talked to me about boys. The girls with whom I had laboured over a papier-mâché game of *A Midsummer Night's Dream*, the gang with whom I had created the fashion house NiftWear (and its lucrative sideline of FIMO earrings) – I ditched them overnight.

There is something profoundly sad about not being able to show people who you really are, and about having friends who don't reflect the inside of you. Of course, every one of us is lots of people over the course of our lives. We try on different selves like outfits for different occasions, and wear different friendships for different outings. There are friendships which only revolve around doing *stuff* together. Friendships which, if you held a mirror up to them, would reflect the people we want to be at a certain moment, not the people we are inside. Some of that exploration is fun. Some of it is painful. But these disparate selves are occasionally only connected to the real *us* by a frail thread, and never more so than during the grub years.

It's lucky, really, that I didn't die in 1992. I don't think people would have had the happiest of memories of me, especially my long-suffering family, who had to put up with the smell of martyred saint wafting around our house (I pretended it was weed, but actually it was mainly joss sticks and the smell of *my pain*). There would have been some hand-wringing about my dying so young, but as a teenage grub I hadn't done much for the world. Something happened, of course, to change things. Call it evolution. Or maybe just growing up. Anyway, I escaped my girls-only torment and went to a different school. Things were better there. I didn't mind wearing my brains on my sleeve so much. Somehow I was accepted into the Cooliverse, even though my wardrobe remained ludicrous. (I must have been the only teenage raver who wore the clothes of a middle-aged woman. Why, when I actually had the body for it, did I not wear actual hot-off-the-streets fashion?)

And then, of course, university, where for the first time things were defined differently. The metric for cool was no longer the number of boy-racers you could kiss, the amount of cider you could drink or whether you had the moves to dance on podiums. Instead, people seemed proud of who they were inside their heads. I met girls who had posters of William Shakespeare on their bedroom walls back home, and were proud of it. Girls who knew who Kant was, even if they pronounced his name cunt (ah, the dangers of being an autodidact). Here it was OK to try hard. It was OK to want to impress the grown-ups. These things contributed to, rather than depleted, your cool status. This was a huge relief for me, though I was overawed too. Who *were* all these confident young people who were both kissable and clever? What rare alchemy had created them? There was an alarming correlation between private schooling and those who emanated this glow. We products of the state school system seemed chippier, more aggressive, less polished, perhaps less comfortable with ourselves. But in any case, here was a place where I could hatch out in safety. With the friction of trying to be something I wasn't removed, and the waves of adolescent hormones calming down, I started to settle into myself.

I was not the only grub who hatched out at around this time. I think of our university bedrooms as a series of little cocoons – messy, sweaty little pits of essay-writing, cigarettes and drunken liaisons from which butterflies eventually emerged. We entered our hatchery in different states; not everyone has their ghoulish period between thirteen and sixteen. Some have it earlier, some much later. And different grubs had different coping strategies. Two I know very well spent their teenage years in hock to a particular brand of Christian evangelism. Now, I have nothing against evangelism (that's not quite true, but let's not go into that now), but religion for them was a mechanism for entering some kind of Cooliverse, since they were excluded from popularity by their nasty little classmates at school. It was a place of certainty and security, while at home a cold war of marital decline reigned. So instead of hanging around their local park drinking White Lightning and lusting after boys doused in cheap aftershave, they directed their unrequited love towards Jesus and his ministers here on earth, handsome young men who played the guitar and whipped up devotion in their female followers. And then they entered the hatchery, there was glasnost (or bust) at home, and the tambourines and guitars no longer seemed quite so necessary.

Another grub arrived with his lank brown hair in curtains, a greasy face and large round spectacles, an oversized Harry Potter without a wand, outwardly full of bonhomie and jollity, inwardly wrestling with whether he wanted to kiss boys or girls. Eventually he decided that boys were his thing, but let's not pretend the hatchling period was easy for him. It was long, messy, and largely private, except for one memorable phone message all his friends received about 4 o'clock one night: 'Ecstasy! Little ginger man! I just want to kiss *all*

the boys. And you! And you!' After that great reve-
lation, things got better.

Some grubs arrived at university appearing to be
butterflies already. Taken in at first by the cool girl
who lived below me, with her leopardskin coat,
London accent and directional hairstyle, I didn't realise until much later that this was her armour — underneath she was every bit as much of an uncertain,
pained little thing as I was; she had just developed
better ways of camouflaging herself than me. You
had to in the big city, I guess. Gradually, over a seem-
ingly endless supply of Jacob's crackers, cheese and
Marlboro Lights, she showed me what was under her
London armour. A brother disabled from birth; a
wealth of anxieties (surprisingly not related to her
directional haircut); a little disability here and there
of her own. Even through her cocoon I could see that
she would end up being my best woman.

I count my time at university as precious not just
because it is where I hatched, but because it is where
I made the friendships that have accompanied me
ever since. I love the company of men. Especially
Billy. But for me there is something special about

female friendship, and it was at university that I began to meet the women who have really mattered to me. I have photos of us back then with wide eyes, big hair and a series of questionable cocktail dresses. We sat around smoking fags, plotting our futures, confident that the world would unfold its riches before us. Like the friends described by Wallace Stegner in *Crossing to Safety* (which is, incidentally, one of the finest novels about friendship I've come across), we 'cut the future into happy stars and circles like little girls making Christmas cookies'.

Together, we were an unstoppable force. Our grubby insecurities and doubts were lost in a haze of cigarette smoke and weak lager, surrendered to the noise of the college jukebox as we shook our cheaply-clad bottoms to the sounds of Nineties girl power. We took our terrible haircuts around the world for adventures; squashed them next to chickens and market ladies in day-long bus journeys; showed them off in the big city in summer temping jobs; flattened them under hats in ski season. When we weren't together, we spent our time writing endless email epistles to one another, recounting tales of our disastrous love lives, moaning about our parents, and generally avoiding the data-entry jobs we were being paid to do in the stifling heat of summer in the city.

While other relationships might define us more – with our parents, partners, or children – for me female friendship has been the steady tick-tock of adult life. And maintaining these friendships over decades was a sign that, finally, I knew who I was inside. The fine thread between myself and *my self* had thickened and settled. I was one with me.

I wonder what it is about women's friendship that is so important. A thousand glossy-magazine articles on the subject haven't helped answer this question. I think conversation is at the heart of it, and it is certainly a truism that there is a lot of verbiage when this particular estate is gathered. Some themes are rather ubiquitous, like a song we keep remixing over the years. Our bodies, whether our thighs look like sausages in leather(ette) leggings, how many sweets have been consumed in the past twenty-four-hour period, whether anyone can see the new-found hairs under our sagging chins. We peer into other people's lives, and yes, we can still be mean girls when we do this. We talk about men, of course. Back in the day, 'Is he into me?' (Usually with an inverse relationship between how into you he was and how much you talked about him.) Now, more mundane: 'How can I teach him to see dirt?' 'Whither the romantic mini-break of old?' I find that parents, and especially mothers, get a decent crack of the lady-chat whip. Children get a look-in too, but not till they are either wanted or have arrived. To the outsider listening in to our discussions, our world might appear limited, narrow, superficial. But listen more carefully. These discussions are just the bacon fat in the stew. They bring things together, keep the friendship well lubricated, make everyday fodder tasty. But without the rest of the conversation that this intimacy permits – the big discussions about life and our place in the world – our friendships would be no more than the dreadful pass-the-time chats had at the back of toddler groups.

I cannot speak here for friendship between men. It is not within my jurisdiction. Billy has been known as the most over-friended man in Britain, and as someone who exercises no judgement at all over his friendships. Perhaps the two are connected. In any event, his smiley face and enjoyment of whisky have gathered around him a bunch of people nearly as interesting, funny and kind as my own friends (some of them I love enough to winkle away and add to my entourage). I don't know what binds him to his menfolk. I don't pretend to understand what they talk about when I'm not there. My suspicion is that they have their own kinds of conversational bacon fat, perhaps revolving around electronic gadgetry, sex and bottom jokes – but like the female equivalent, it is just the grease in the engine of the more profound discussions.

These discussions are the other side of friendship. The conversations and the memories and the fun you have together permit you to reveal the weak, scared vulnerable self that emerges every now and again. My second operation – the one I had to chop the pesky tumours out of my liver, six months after my diagnosis and my first op – was tough. It took place in a shiny, cancer-defeating factory in Houston, because Billy's careful research had shown that it had the best chance of successfully ridding me of cancer. We spent nearly a month there, and Stateside I was the glummest of glum girls. The operation depleted me in a way I could never have imagined. Agonisingly painful. Full of complications and miserable rehospitalisations. I finally returned home feeling drained of everything, including optimism. This was ironic, as post-operation I was in a better place, statistically, than I'd been since my original diagnosis six months previously: my odds of surviving the next five years leapt (briefly) from 6 per cent to 50 per cent. And yet for me it was the darkest part of the night. Maybe because everyone breathed a sigh of relief, and thought the crisis was over. Maybe because I was physically weaker than I've ever been. I don't know why, but for several months there was a loneliness to my sadness which I hadn't experienced before.

In that kind of situation, there are two options. The first is to battle through on your own. To grit your teeth, put your head down, and say things will be better tomorrow (whenever tomorrow comes). I call this the Scarlett O'Hara; it is a noble approach, one I've taken before, and one that I know appeals to the proud, quiet, maybe more masculine side of all of our natures. But I chose the second option, which was to write a list of my best women, and ask them to come and help. We sat in the garden. The tulips were out, and I howled snottily on their shoulders in a way I hadn't before. After that I told them about my fears and loneliness, and how bloody awful everything had been. Then things got better.

Not long before the Nuisance, my fear had been that the really good times were over for these wonderful friendships. Thirty-somethings with children, jobs and partners to attend to, we were no longer as available to one another as we used to be. While I might wish we all lived in some kind of giant child-rearing commune, that isn't the case. Friendships survive on scraps of time and emails, squeezed between the rest of life, and very often conducted thousands of miles apart. We live off well-trodden stories, the space in our lives for making new memories mostly taken up by family and work, where the real drama happens. The odd dinner, more often a cup of tea balanced precariously over a baby's head while we converse, but never enough time for the real stuff, or for new adventures together. I always hoped there would be time for that again, if only in the Home for Neglected Mothers of Sons in which we would end up in our dotage. But now it seems that I won't be checking into that particular nursing home. All the same, there is a happy postscript to this story, at least in Nuisance land. As one of these wise women says, quoting Mike Tyson, 'Everyone has a plan until they get punched in the face.' We all had our plans. Our paths criss-crossed as we got on with life, friendships always there when they needed to be picked up. But then my family got punched in the face, far earlier and far harder than we could have expected, and our plans melted away. Suddenly time was carved out for friendship again. So cancer has given as well as it has taken – though perhaps it is more accurate to say that our friendships take from it what they can, a collective two fingers to all the Nuisance stands for.

I have spent so much of the past few years under the spell of chemotherapy, existing in a half-life where every fortnight is split into seven days of misery and seven days of life. Aside from (temporarily) taming my cancer, the other benefit of having this wicked set of toxins poured into me is that I see more of my resplendent friends from around the world than I have done for years. I am accompanied into the chemo ward. I am visited at home. This is lucky, because 'therapy' is a complete misnomer for the cruel concoction of drugs which is infused into my bloodstream in an attempt to keep me alive. But it has to be done: as Claudius puts it in *Hamlet*, 'Diseases desperate grown by desperate appliance are relieved, Or not at all.'

I imagine my own desperate appliance as a particularly inept vigilante marauding through my body on the hunt for cancer cells. He shoots – he kills! Oh no. More often than not, what he has slaughtered is a perfectly healthy cell just going about its taste-creating, nausea-controlling, body-hydrating business. Chemo is all about this clumsy collateral damage and how to manage it: hence the phalanx of steroids, anti-nausea pills and so on, each of which brings its own wicked side-effects. But what I hadn't reckoned with was the mental stuff. My vigilante seems particularly adept at shooting down serotonin, so that for a few days the chemicals replace my soul with a shrivelled black void. With each cycle the physical and emotional scar tissue deepens. I elect to return, but only just.

If I wasn't accompanied by my very own Terracotta Army of friends, returning to the chemo ward would be harder. They make things bearable. They understand the little things. That, even facing death, for me (like Hillary Clinton and her scrunchies) it's *still* all about the hair (and lack thereof). That seeing the oncologist is easier when I'm in a tough-girl leopard-skin coat with a slick of bright red lippy. That though my heart's desire cannot be granted, that doesn't mean I don't desire stuff. The ancient Egyptians had it right – the urge to accumulate beautiful treasures increases the closer you get to death; and I intend to go into the afterlife looking polished, surrounded by the luxury goods given to me by the best women. They understand the big things too: how I need to live in Technicolor in the time I can. They plan holidays. We visit Paris in the rain. They take me to the newest restaurants, and send me extravagant bunches of flowers and richly scented candles so that in the evening I can draw the curtains and pretend that everything is *just fine*.

I sometimes sit in my chair, too tired to move, too brain-dead to read or write. With my eyes closed, I feel a pleasant weight pressing on my shoulders. It is the weight of all the time Billy and I have had with our friends, enveloping me like a heavy blanket. They are brave, these people. They were there the day after I was diagnosed, uninvited, hugging Billy and regaling me with tales of dreadful in-laws that made me laugh so much my new scar throbbed through the morphine. They are there when I come out of the claustrophobic scanning machines, squeezing my hand as I fretfully try to interpret every look the radiographers give each other. They arrive at our door with elaborate dishes for lunch, and then stay to do the washing up. Part of the reassuring weight I feel from these friendships comes from the discussions we have had about Afterwards. These are the kind of friends who want to be in my children's lives forever. The kind of friends who will buy seven-seater cars to ferry them around as well as their own families. The kind of friends who will tell stories of Mummy long after she's gone. The kind of friends who will pick Billy up when gritting his teeth and saying tomorrow will be a better day just doesn't cut it.

I'm not leaving my children much in the way of a big house, sumptuous gardens or (I wish) Austen's magical ten thousand a year. But I am leaving an estate of people who have cherished me, and who will cherish them forever. Ah, Yeats, you old Irish soak, you were right:

> Think where man's glory most begins and ends
> And say my glory was I had such friends.

3

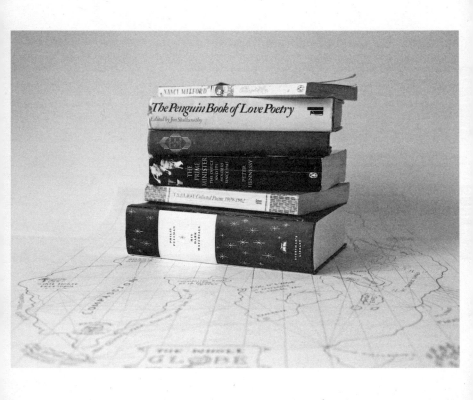

The Landscape of Your Mind

'Understand this,' said Xaphania. 'Dust is not a constant. There's not a fixed quantity that has always been the same. Conscious beings make Dust – they renew it all the time, by thinking and feeling and reflecting, by gaining wisdom and passing it on. And if you help everyone else in your worlds to do that, by helping them to learn and understand about themselves and each other and the way everything works, and by showing them how to be kind instead of cruel, and patient instead of hasty, and cheerful instead of surly, and above all how to keep their minds open and free and curious ... Then they will renew enough to replace what is lost through one window.'

PHILIP PULLMAN, *THE AMBER SPYGLASS*

I am a woman of words married to a man of science. Curiosity reigns in our household. I am certain that if my darling boys can retain a fraction of the inquisitiveness they possess at five, they will have the key to a limitless intellectual hinterland that will accompany them forever. It's simple, really. Inside our heads are vast, uncharted miracles of squidgy grey matter. Somehow, this unguent tissue allows us to be conscious – to think and feel and imagine. Though it is bounded by the bony limits of our skull, the stuff inside is limitless. What a thing your brain is. To paraphrase Sherlock Holmes, the rest of you, your body, is really just an appendix to it. It is the bit of you that *is*, that makes you who you are. You need to tend it, nurture it with questions and answers, clear away the weeds once in a while. You can let it get parched and dry for a while; the green shoots will still be there, hibernating, waiting for you to give them a long cool drink, but leave it arid too long at your peril. And it is yours, only yours. It is portable, light as a feather, and you can carry it even when everything else is too heavy.

What is the landscape of *your* mind? Broad open plains, or deep river valleys? What nurtures and feeds it? I can show you mine; but first I will tell you about Billy's, because laying his hinterland out next to mine is like travelling from the Kenyan savanna to the Appalachian mountains, so different are our internal geographies. Billy grew up in Belfast, a child of the Eighties, a teen of the Nineties. Things were quieter, better, there when he was growing up than they had been for his five elder siblings, but the Troubles were still his normal. 'The Troubles' is such a very Northern Irish way of describing a long, horrible and violent time. One of his sisters remembers her weekly trip to the library with her dad not only because it lit up her blossoming imagination, but because one day the place was suddenly full of British soldiers, and she remembers her dad pushing her to the ground, telling her to keep calm, and then when the shouting and the guns went quiet, running all the way home with her in his arms.

For Billy, the Troubles had a positive and powerful legacy: an escape into the wider world, which set his little mind on fire. Aged eleven, he became one of the 'Project Children' (what a name), a group of Protestant and Catholic mini-teens sent to summer with affluent families in America. Designed as horizon-expanding inter-religious bonding, it was also waistline-expanding, and the place Billy had his first kiss, with a Protestant girl called Kelly. He was exposed to plenty, and liked it so much he went back every summer for four years. Plenty in what people had, plenty in what they ate, plenty in how they thought. He saw in Americans an ease with the idea of the big wide world, an assumption of their privileged place in it, of their ability to do whatever it was they set their hearts on. After that, Andersonstown Road might be home, but it wouldn't ever be enough. When his big brother went off to do his Masters at Cambridge, Billy visited with his parents. Aged fourteen, he sat in his shiny LA Raiders tracksuit underneath the statue of Isaac Newton in Trinity College chapel and decided that he would be a scientist. And that is how things ended up, against the odds.

Young Billy's mental landscape, formed by those years in Belfast and his time in the land of plenty, is recognisably that of big Billy: he is an explorer of interior worlds, pushing the boundaries of his mind by charting, measuring and mapping what he finds around him. The first stirrings of this exploration came with the arrival of a microscope into his life when he was eight or nine, through which a different side of the world was opened up. Then, the ritual dissection and reassembly of any and all electronic objects. Getting the hang of Airfix model aeroplanes, reeking of glue and causing his father to worry that he had a secret sniffing habit. All this, and more, went to make up the man I have known, whose relentless curiosity never fails to make me feel lazy. In a decade he has worked his way through British and American politics; the workings of the European Union (this in an attempt to make conversation during our early courtship); the philosophy of science; philosophy more generally, with a particular interest in the Stoics; the inner workings of Microsoft Excel, Salesforce and a million other technological advances which will be ancient history by the time you read this; oncology; and now, poor man, palliative care. For Billy, to understand something is to have mastery over it. Life is uncontrollable, and messy, but looking it square in the eye, buying a book about it and then working out what his own mind makes of it all – well, that is his way of dealing with things.

Billy has been my chief scientific officer, navigating this new terrain of disease and taking on the medical establishment with knowledge of his own. He has sifted through impenetrable cancer journals to understand the latest treatment options and clinical trials. He has spoken to medical experts all around the world. He sat down with a professor of game theory in Cambridge to try to understand the tyranny of the statistics that faced us. He did this because there was a long period after my diagnosis and first operation when the way ahead was not clear. We had hopes, then, of a complete recovery, if I could only get the pesky tumours out of my liver. But who knew what the best way to do that was? There was a plethora of views. It was like walking along the edge of a precipice, each tiny step potentially edging us to a place of greater safety, but with the risk of tumbling over at any point. The problem was (and is) that we never knew what safety looked like. Although we searched for a sign saying 'This way, to avoid the end of the world,' we couldn't see one. And the doctors kept introducing us to dreadful new words like 'equipoise' – that is, they didn't know either. But what power to be able to decide, to have a choice. What a sense of agency it gave back to us when we needed it most. In the old days, we would simply have been folded into the huge, benign arms of the NHS: a plan would have been made for us by the well-meaning state. I might not even have been told I had cancer, because people weren't, back then, in case the awareness of the C word alone sent them into a terminal decline. But things are different now, and we patients are encouraged to make decisions for ourselves. It has been hard to navigate this world with our imperfect knowledge, but Billy's forensic approach has provided the tools with which to chart this strange new terrain. For him, it's like the King James Bible. Being able to read it for yourself, in your own tongue, gives you power. Having it read to you makes you passive, and kills the questions that keep your brain alive.

* * *

And how does the land lie in my mind? We have established that it is not moved by numbers, statistics, or the laws of physics. The science of my disease bores me. I am spending my last days writing this book. I am about words. Words are how I understand the world – I read, therefore I am. They are more than a means of expression and a conduit to knowledge: they are the way I see beauty. I have no musical ear. I like art, and have stood transfixed before paintings, but nothing stirs my soul like language. Words provide entertainment. Solace. Space. Excitement. All of this has always been true, but somewhere along the way things got blurred, and it is only in these past few luminous years that it has become clear to me again.

From the window in our attic bedroom, you can see the spreading branches and fine, silvery leaves of our neighbours' eucalyptus tree, incongruously big in the small, square garden of a suburban terraced house. This room is where I convalesced when I first got sick, where I now sit when the rest of the house below vibrates with noise and energy. I watch the leaves dance, and shards of brown bark fly off in the wind. I can imagine the particular, bitter smell of eucalyptus as I sit cocooned from the world.

As my body healed in those early weeks after my first diagnosis, parts of me which had been hibernating for years began to wake up. I started to read again. But I could not bear very much reality, so I read books from my childhood. I began to identify with the invalid heroines. I was too jolly to be Mary Lennox from *The Secret Garden*. Too bossy and not quite sickly enough to be Beth from *Little Women* – when it came down to it, I idolised Jo above all the other March sisters. Not because Laurie loved her first and best, but because she loved words as I did. As I read, I felt the stirrings of a voice inside me. The voice of a bookish ten-year-old girl, who had planned one day to be poet laureate, writing dreadful poetry (sample: *It's Saturday, hip hip hooray!/The day that* Bunty *comes my way*), but feeling singular satisfaction as she learned to craft words so that they gave perfect shape and form to what she felt inside. The little voice inside grew louder and more confident. For the first time since my anguished, diary-writing teenage years I had something that demanded to be written about. Left to my own devices, the rebirth of this little voice might have led to a round-robin email every month and a few pathetic poems. But the man in my life is a technological early-adopter, and by this stage Billy had already started two blogs. Neither had taken the world by storm, but that was perhaps because their subject-matter was Excel. Nonetheless, I took his advice, and nineteen days after my diagnosis I posted my first blog. Partly as a way of making my voice heard, and connecting my attic room to a bigger world out there. Partly as a way of owning – and challenging – this new cancer lexicon which I felt had nothing to do with me. Partly just because amidst all the talk of death, the only thing I felt I could do was create something new. I wrote (I write) myself into existence to stop existence being taken from me.

I write because I read, and books have accompanied me all my life. When we moved back to England from the Middle East, I joined a library and got an adult reader's ticket so I could take home eight books a week rather than the meagre child-ration of four. I would sit with my back up against the radiator, head resting on the green velvet curtains in the basement of our gold-stoned house in Bath, reading and reading. All of Agatha Christie's murder mysteries by the time I was eleven, in a crime-fighting fetish that began with the Titian-haired delights of Nancy Drew. An obsession with Greek myths, where I was Artemis, goddess of the moon, an ambitiously physical role model for my bookish pre-teen self. In books I journeyed to fantasy lands – Narnia, Green Ginger, Oz, Ingary, Trebond, Brisingamen, Middle Earth. Then historical novels, falling in love with Elizabeth I through the many great works of Jean Plaidy. (Who cares about the reality? Liz will always be my heroine.) And later, in Manley Hopkins' 'towery city and branchy between towers', ranging through the full canon of English literature, some under duress from my tutors (Tennyson, Richardson), some through my own free will (Milton, Shakespeare, Austen, Langland, Chaucer).

Milton taught me how words could change worlds, of their political potency. He wrote in a time when the printing press was still a relatively new technology, and for the first time words and ideas could be spread around the populace rapidly and without relying on the physical presence of the speaker. For Milton, words were alive – 'Books are not absolutely dead things, but doe contain a potencie of life in them to be as active as that soule was whose progeny they are; nay they do preserve as in a violl the purest efficacie and extraction of that living intellect that bred them.' (I trust that something of this potencie of life will bring me alive when my children read this.) Milton argued for 'the liberty to know, to utter, and to argue freely', saying that we should be trusted to be responsible, to read what we choose and to make what we will of it – which of course is precisely the luxury I have had, unlike so many in the world now and in the past. In that towery city I also learned to love poetry, though I can't pretend to understand it. Poetry just *is*, and I sometimes wonder if trying to grasp it too closely removes some of its power. I get what Archibald MacLeish says – 'A poem should not mean/But be.'

If there is a justification for the extravagance that is a three-year English degree, this is it. Reading is an experience by which we connect ourselves to what we are, to this magnificent, awful life, in which the same grooves are being scored over and over again in different times and tongues. It is about how you experience humanity. As John Berger said, 'The poet places language beyond the reach of time; or, more accurately, the poet approaches language as if it were an assembly point, where time has no finality, where time itself is encompassed and constrained.' Life, death, love, loss, war, God in the detail, men are like buses, they fuck us up our mum and dad, and so on. The whole of human experience is there in the language we have created. Words allow you not just to express yourself, but to become someone else, for a moment. The capacity to feel empathy, to understand others, to have an imagination – this is what it means to be human, and this is what reading provides. Ian McEwan put it well: 'Cruelty is a failure of imagination.' If you can imagine, you can empathise. You can exist in someone else's world. You can explore your terrors and your dreams.

Because of this, I like to think that my wordy mental landscape has a purpose, other than my own pleasure. Reading has allowed me to imagine myself into the great expanse of mankind; to experience other people's suffering and their joy, unconstrained by the time I live in, unbound from my own relative affluence and good luck. Accessing other people's stories ignited a spark in my young mind which I now recognise as empathy. I freely admit that some-times this spark is fuelled by a rubbernecking 'There but for the grace of God' fear, but on my better days this becomes compassion, an awareness of my connectedness to and responsibility for the world around me. In the same way, I know that people will want to read my story because it takes them to the edge of their fears about dying young, leaving the people who need them. I am grateful for that capac-ity, for the compassion it ignites in others as well as me. We are all voyeurs in our fear.

I look for different words at different times, words to explain the world I find around me. In the past few years I have read all I can on the subject of illness. It is strange but fascinating that so little is written about sickness and death, given their universality as part of the human experience. 'There is no decent literature on how to die,' says the strident Charity Lang on her deathbed in Wallace Stegner's *Crossing to Safety*. Virginia Woolf is even more lucid in her essay 'On Being Ill':

> Considering how common illness is, how tremendous the spiritual change it brings, how astonishing, when the lights of health go down, the undiscovered countries that are then disclosed, what wastes and deserts of the soul a slight attack of influenza brings to view, what precipices and lawns sprinkled with bright flowers a little rise of temperature reveals ... it is strange indeed that illness has not taken its place with love and battle and jealousy among the prime themes of literature.

Perhaps the reason for this is clear. Like childbirth, when it is over, illness is erased swiftly from memory. Emily Dickinson understood the trance-like forgetting that follows trauma: 'There is a pain – so utter/It swallows substance up/Then covers the Abyss with Trance/So Memory can step/Around – across – upon it'. And if it is not over; well, what follows is death, and the grave is hardly conducive to the creative spirit.

There are beginning to be exceptions – brilliant, funny writing in what I think of as the Cancer Canon: public figures, journalists and writers who approach their own death and those of the people they love with words, because that is what they have been used to doing with the rest of their lives. They have an elegance, providing insight which I have gloomily devoured, looking for wisdom on how to end my days. Emily Rapp, an American writer who lost her little boy to Tay-Sachs Disease, says: 'We all avoid death – we don't want to see it, talk about it or think about it. But digging into the experience of loss is not only deeply profound but artistically, at some points, absolutely electric. People want (and sometimes encourage) the griever to numb it or erase it or at the very least ignore it, and all a writer can think to do is pull it closer and dig in her fingernails and hang on.' Writing like this provides a flash of brilliance amongst an otherwise unrewarding sea of misery memoirs. Never (says the woman with a blog about cancer) spend time on cancer blogs. An evening spent morbidly reading other people's death stories is guaranteed to send me into a spiral of despair – at my own miserable demise, and at the godawful writing which the internet licenses in the name of sharing the human experience.

I have told the stories of two hinterlands, in the hope that they will help you decipher your own. But I think I must end this chapter with a warning. It is too easy, as an adult, to let life rush past with its business of succeeding, working, consuming, rearing. All of that can be joyful and fulfilling, I grant you. But it is so, so easy in the rush of life to neglect your inner world. I know mine was dead for many years, squeezed between work and achieving *stuff* and my darling little ones – it's a choice I made, and gladly. But one of the unexpected blessings of illness is that it has given me time to tend my mind again. And how I have enjoyed this, how much pleasure and solace it has provided even when things have been at their bleakest. I can see my own hinterland, and that means I can see other people's too. Conversations have become more than merely transactional exchanges ('How are you?', 'What are you up to?'). I talk about the things that really matter. My voice – quiet for too long – roars. Even as one little room becomes my everywhere, I roam the wide plains of my mind. When I finally stop reading, I will be read to, departing this world as I arrived in it, with the sound of stories echoing in my ears.

4

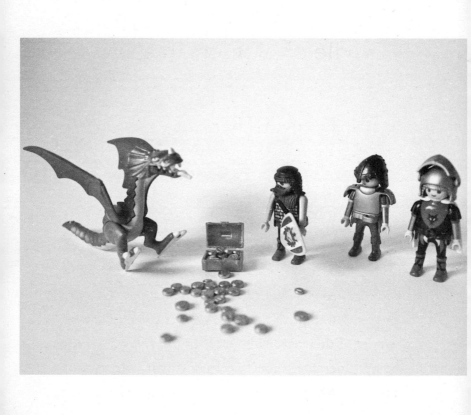

A Pile of Golden Treasure

Right, like a well-done sum.
A clean slate, with your own face on

SYLVIA PLATH, 'YOU'RE'

Is there ever a time when you are prepared to die? While I am having chemotherapy I look across the room at people in their fifties, sixties, and wonder if they are on the way out, or on the cusp of a cure. I wonder if they have kids. I feel angry with them for being older than me. I feel angry with them for surviving when I won't. And then I am angry with myself. Who am I to imagine their stories, or to say that my suffering is worse than theirs? I have no idea what their deal is. But then the visceral part of me which gave birth to twin boys shouts 'Bollocks.' There is an immutable fact here – my children exist. I am leaving them too young, and it is wrong. So I sometimes try to bargain with the fates. Give me five years. No, give me ten, till they are fifteen. No, twenty years is what I need. Then I would go quietly, and without a fuss. But that won't happen. I'm not even going to get another year. I am left trying to make sense of what it means to be a mother now, and what the future might be like for them without me.

Love set my babies going like a pair of fat gold watches. They popped out on 12 May 2009 in an operating theatre in Cambridge. The last few weeks of pregnancy had been uncomfortable. I was vast, like an ocean liner. People laughed at me on the street. When I lay in a hot bath, the two unborn boys writhed around my insides, kicking one another like two trapped aliens. Oscar came out first, and a minute later Isaac, lifted out of my open tummy by a gentleman in a green gown and a silly hat. They slept next to me, curled up together in a Perspex cot as we spent our first nights together on the maternity ward. They slept, and I stayed awake, fuelled by crazy happy hormones and the terror of this new-found responsibility. In those early days, some people asked me how it was possible to have enough love to share between two babies at exactly the same time. They asked me if I had a favourite twin. These people were usually the parents of a single child; they couldn't imagine their love stretching to another. But some of them went on to have more children themselves, and then they understood. They understood that the amount of love I have for my children is elastic, infinite; and at the same time, profoundly different – because you love your children for who they are, whatever they are.

When Oscar first popped out I loved this dark-haired, violet-eyed little being. Personality shows itself early on, and I was and am bewitched by his character, which is so his own, though at the same time he reminds me of Billy, and of Billy's own father. From early on, his concentration amazed me. His ability to focus on things, to want to know them utterly. First came farm machinery (with a particular specialisation in combine harvesters), then

Transformers, then venomous animals, and now computer games. Aged three, when he didn't have the playthings he wanted, he learned to 'put his imagination on things', to transform an old toy car into a superhero vehicle. He will never be bounded by a nutshell.

Isaac is blond and quick to tan, his olive skin the opposite of Oscar's dark Irish looks. I adore how he lives in the present, impatient and excited to know the world. He listens intently to other people's conversations – adults, children – desperate to be inside our minds, and to let us inside his own wild imagination and furious curiosity. Most of the time he is ebullient, physical, showing off his baby-boy sixpack as he literally climbs the walls of our house; then his mood changes, rain coming in like an April shower, and we retreat upstairs to read about Narnia, little Isaac safe in my arms but far away in his imagination.

They were always such separate little beings, my two boys, their difference eliciting surprise from strangers who somehow expected twins to be clones. Who knows whether the little people they are at five will reflect the big people they are at twenty-five, forty-five, sixty-five. The last thing I want to do is 'fix' them now, their personalities in opposition to one another; or one twin like Mummy, one twin like Daddy. It is too easy to typecast them; the truth is they each bear a little of me, a little of Billy, and a lot of themselves. And each of them carved out his own space in my heart, a space which fits him exactly.

Billy had made our little house on Bateman Street perfect on the day we brought them home from hospital. Of those early weeks, I remember two things vividly. The first is being utterly and completely nuts, deranged by this new-found mother-love and wicked sleep deprivation. The second is taking them to the Cambridge Botanic Garden for the first time. Billy proudly wheeled the double buggy. We constantly checked that they were still breathing. We took photos underneath Isaac Newton's (big Isaac's) apple tree. We have been there so many times since, but that was the first in our new formation, our perfect nuclear family. Oscar was mesmerised at an early age by trees; he would watch the leaves sway overhead contemplatively, big eyes in his wide moon face. Isaac loved people. As he learned to hold his head up he followed our voices around the room; humans were fascinating, and sleep was to be resisted at all costs. He had to be fooled into it, lulled off before he realised it was happening.

Then they grew. They grew and they grew into fat, jolly little babies. I stayed at home for the first nine months. It wasn't easy. Wrangling two little bodies in and out of nappies, buggies, coats, was hard physical labour. They were full of energy. We partitioned our front room, half of it enclosed behind a large metal gate. This was solely so that I could go to the toilet or make a cup of tea without an escape being made. But it meant that when I left the room, they would pull themselves up on the bars and hang from them, wailing until I came back. Better that, I thought, than hurtling down the stairs or trying to shut one another in the washing machine. Those were happy days, untroubled. I managed motherhood, though not always with good grace. I trained the boys in the art of watching television early on, eager for some time when they were neither biting one another nor requiring my constant presence to play tractors. This is to say I wasn't a perfect mother, even in those golden times. I was frustrated, cross, haphazard and always tired. Eventually I went back to work for half the week. I flew off to Africa every month. But I was there, and we were together, and they were mine.

There is nothing so elemental as the love of a mother for a child. I think of it like an Anglo-Saxon góld-hòrd (my schooling in Anglo-Saxon poetry finally proving useful by furnishing me with this beautiful metaphor), a weighty treasure store heavy with adoration, and with worry. Worry is the currency of my love, because worry is *just what I do*, and how love manifests itself in my world. Worry for them now, worry for the future. I have tried hard to pass on only the adoration, because little shorts have such small pockets, and carrying all my concerns around would make it very hard to climb the highest trees and slide down the sheerest drops.

I was first diagnosed with cancer when the boys were three and a half. They have grown up with my illness. It has shaped our lives, the mother I am and the father Billy is and will be. I don't know how much they will remember from 'Before'. In the early days, certainly, they knew there was a difference in me. When I came back from hospital with my 'tummy hurt' they had to be *deli-cat*. I couldn't carry them around on my back like little princes. Worst of all, we couldn't go swimming together. This has been the greatest blow, because Billy is a scaredy-cat and I am a water nymph. A few months after my first operation, we drove past the outdoor paddling pool at Lammas Land and Oscar said, apropos of nothing, 'That's where we used to go before your tummy hurt, Mummy.' Later on, in my interlude of wellness, I tried and failed to cycle them both up a hill in our Dutch bike, and Isaac explained loudly to passers-by that 'Mummies are weak but daddies are strong, that's why she has to push the bike.' I snapped back that it was only *their* mummy who was weak; the rest of the female sex are quite as robust as the daddies.

They were meant to grow up with a sibling. From the moment they were born, in the back of my mind was the idea that someday they would have a sister (I attribute this expectation to a childhood fantasy in which I was the naughty little sister to two rambunctious, smart, cheeky older brothers). But fictitious little baby Josie ceased to exist the moment I was diagnosed, another part of our future that melted away overnight. Chemotherapy fried my ovaries and tipped me from childbearing thirty-something into the thin-haired, SAGA-holidaying, all-that's-behind-me menopausal bracket in a matter of months. So, Plan Josie became Josie the baby ghost. Now she is a little girl who grows older only in a parallel world, the kind you find by accident at the back of a wardrobe, or through a crease in time. I think about her often. She is true and real in another life I'm having, somewhere else.

I don't know if my real, live children – my darling Knights – can sense that the difference in me is not merely physical. It isn't just that I am in bed so much after my 'sleepy medicine'. I am different now. I am careful, diligent, emotional, fretful, where I used to be careless, disorganised, energetic. Now I only want to be the good guy, and Billy is left to do all the crappy bits of parenting: the tooth-brushing, the discipline, the hair-brushing. I cuddle too tightly. I cherish the time spent watching ninja cartoons together before school, when I should be wishing it away so I can get on with work or the washing or something more important. I do not pretend this makes me a better mother. I think the opposite, actually, and I hope they remember something of the woman who was around before the spectre of leaving drained away her easy confidence in parenting. But now, at least, I am here. These are still good times, strangely wonderful times, and we are closer now than ever, we three. Emily Rapp wrote of the same tightening link between her and her dying son, whose forever-soft baby hair she celebrates in *The Still Point of the Turning World*: 'The world was strange and jagged but we were together in it, spinning inside some powerful centrifugal force that is the bond between parent and child.'

I know what it will be like when I deteriorate; I know because I remember only too well what it felt like after my operations. When the veil of real pain and weakness comes down, their little tousled heads drift away. Pain redirects my limited energy towards myself. I can be in touching distance of them, but so far away. Unable to feign interest in their latest Lego models, unwilling to read to them, no longer able to explore the boundaries of their little hinterlands. This is what it will be like at the end. I will drift away from them without a choice, because my body will make it so. That helps, in a funny way, because the thought of saying goodbye while I am still able to hold their hands tightly is impossible.

Everyone in our orbit thinks about the boys more than anything else. When I talk about dying, which I do a lot, and with what I suspect is alarming pragmatism, the question people ask me is, 'How are the boys?' I know what they really mean, even though they don't voice it. They want to know if the boys know I am going to die. They want to know how I feel about leaving my children when they are so young. The truth is, the boys don't know I am going to die. Not yet, anyway. We will tell them when it is imminent, because small brains deal in the present, not the future, and there is no point in putting the nightmare into their lives before it has to be there.

They have enough to worry about with the zombies that nibble their toes in the night. When Isaac asked, 'Will you still be alive when I'm a grown-up, Mummy?', I fudged the answer. But I rehearse the conversation we will have to have with them in my mind every day. How will they react? With tears, or denial? How can I comfort them when I will be falling apart myself?

And as for me – well, I can bear anything except leaving them. I find life hard to let go of. I hate the way my body is going to ruin. I want to run again. If I can't run, I want to walk, to climb mountains with fresh streams running through wooded valleys, to see the snow on high peaks, to swim in clear seas, to dive off hot rocks into cold water. But I would gladly spend the rest of my life confined to one room if it meant I could spend it with my family. I was told a story of one small boy who, when told his mummy wasn't going to get better from her cancer, didn't understand that this meant she would die. He thought she would just continue to be ill-mummy, in bed forever. I am not beyond wishing that were a possibility for us.

But I find I am able to rationalise even the leaving of my beloveds. I still can't bear it, but I can find a way to make it the best it can be. Because what we are given is time – time to make memories, time to say goodbye, time for me to write this so that when they are grown they will have something real of me to know. More than anything, I can rationalise it because although there isn't a world where I am there to commiserate when they fail their driving tests, to make an embarrassing mother-of-the-groom speech at their weddings, to coo over their babies, there is no world where I haven't been there for the first five years of their lives. I know without a doubt what it means for them to have been surrounded by my treasure chest of love in these precious early years. It provided security, even before they could register their surroundings. Now it is what makes them confident in their little world, able to go to school and make friends and explore the unknown. It is gold in their bank for the rest of their lives. Even without the Mummy-Master of the góld-hòrd, their accounts will remain full of the treasure we have checked in early on. And conversely, if they had not had this security, this love, at such an early age, there is no repaying it. In this, at least, they are luckier than so many children in the world.

Of course, I think all the time about what life will be like when our family is three, not four. There will be a lot of testosterone, tempers and computer games. The washing basket will reek of BOY. Because I am nothing if not a control freak, I am trying to plan life well into the ever-after. There is an instruction manual to make the house tick. Various surrogate mothers have been versed in where to buy school trousers and when to get eyes tested. Someone will make sure the sheets are washed every now and again. These last months have seen a flurry of reverse-nesting, home-making for the dying, as I prepare the house for an eternity without me, as if looking down from the afterlife and seeing stained old carpets and a crumbling bathroom would eternally shame me when their friends come round to play. I want our kitchen to remain full of messy artwork, jars of tadpoles, and people laughing around the battered old table. I dread our home becoming a cold, sad place laden with unhappy memories. I can't let that happen. Anyway, I will still be there. I am a part of the four walls around. The colours are my colours. The sofas are the ones I curl up on to sleep like an oversize family cat. The pictures are the ones Billy and I chose over the years, memories of places we went on our endless, lazy, pre-baby walks around London, New York, Paris.

In thinking about Afterwards, I have sought out the stories of people who lost parents at an early age. How I wish there weren't so many stories. But they are everywhere. I am dumbstruck by the ability of these friends, these friends of friends, these strangers, to share their pasts with me. Of course it is impossible to generalise. Of course. But these people are All Right. In fact, many of them are far more than All Right; they love with all their hearts. They live in the moment, because they know that is all we can do. They cherish their own families. There is something in these people's tales that made me begin to hope that my family would be All Right, too. First, this, from a lovely young woman who is also an accomplished diplomat:

> I sometimes don't know what to do with the strength of feeling I have for my children. Like you, I'm messy at motherhood: sometimes I get it wrong, sometimes I get frustrated, sometimes I overcompensate. So I wanted to share this with you: somehow my mum got it really right (no such thing, I know; it's either right or not. But you know what I mean). She didn't leave me letters, or wishes for what I'd grow up like. She didn't get me to make her promises. She just mothered me. Wrapped me in that golden yet invisible security blanket of knowing I was loved. And it was more than enough. I lost her many years ago. And there ought to be some scientific equation that means the years we had together were only enough to see me through a certain number of years into adulthood. But that hasn't been my experience. The trove was well enough stocked just through the fierceness of her love for me.

Then this, from a man who lives on the other side of the world:

> Many people wonder how their children will handle milestones if they are not around. I hope that I can shed some light on this, as I have gone through nearly every major milestone with just my mum. Graduation, birthdays, weddings, births, monster-truck shows – the big events. And here's the thing. It's hard, but there's a bittersweet aspect to every milestone. You can take stock and you have a moment in your own heart where quietly, on your own, you can simply reflect. You learn to try and soak up everything that you can, because you, more than most people, know that things don't last. I have always tried to make time and drink it all in, and to make sure others are drinking it in with me. I like to stop and make sure that it's in my mind forever.

And finally this, from the best woman of my best woman, when told by her potential new stepmother than she didn't want to 'replace her real mum'.

I had to hide my confusion and laughter, it was like someone telling me that you could replace fire with wind. As far as I was aware, the position of biologically giving birth to me, nursing me and giving me my eyes, sense of humour and apple figure wasn't up for grabs. No one could ever tell me they loved me like she did, and no one ever really needed to again, because it was my grounding, my bedrock. Just because I wasn't told it every hour again, didn't mean I didn't feel it encircle me.

None of this changes the fact that I don't have enough time to celebrate my babies' hair (or their fingers, toes, dastardly love of plots, fart jokes and sweeties). But knowing that what we have already had matters does help. And so does knowing that I will be around – in the walls of our house, in memories, in my friends, in the words I love and in the words I write. I'm gone. But at the same time I'm not, and never will be.

5

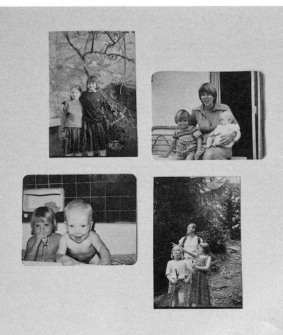

The Original Four-Square

And slowly, Harry looked into the faces of the other people in the mirror and saw other pairs of green eyes like his, other noses like his, even a little old man who looked as though he had Harry's knobbly knees – Harry was looking at his family, for the first time in his life.

The Potters smiled and waved at Harry and he stared hungrily back at them, his hands pressed flat against the glass as though he was hoping to fall right through it and reach them. He had a powerful kind of ache inside him, half joy, half terrible sadness.

J.K. ROWLING, *HARRY POTTER AND*
THE PHILOSOPHER'S STONE

It is early evening. I am on a rickety bicycle, with my sister Jo riding next to me. We are just outside the town of Hoi An, a beautiful, painted place of low-rise buildings, small temples, cool verandas and thousands upon thousands of tailors, working fine Vietnamese silk into the latest designs from *Vogue* for crowds of greedy tourists. The road to the beach is flat and even, surrounded by green paddy fields, crowded with people going in the same direction as us. When we reach the sand, there are no other back-packers there. Our Western faces are lost in a sea of Vietnamese families rolling up their trousers after work or school, paddling in the ocean, sitting in makeshift beach cafés enjoying a Fanta and a plate of fried soft-shell crab.

We sit in the evening sun, my sister and I. We have separately been wending our way around the world, planning to meet up in this lovely country, thousands of miles from home. Jo has been working in Saigon for six months; I have been journeying towards her from India, following the monsoon. We have arrived on this beach by very different paths, but we come from the same place. Nature and nurture have brought us here, not accident. We travel on inherited passports: Mum and Dad, who spent the first years of their marriage in the shadow of the Alborz mountains in pre-revolutionary Tehran; Grandpa, with his wartime exploits in India and Burma; our Aunt Alison, who has seen more of Africa than I ever will. Jo and I talk about family, catching up on each other's news from home. I am reminded by this iridescent memory of a perfect evening that the family I come from – the two-by-two of a nuclear family, the solid four-square – is as indivisible as the family I have created. For twenty-odd years, mother, father and sister were the permanent features of my landscape, and I of theirs. And this original four-square is being hewn apart by the bloody Nuisance too.

Of course, the ties between us four Grosses have loosened since the days when Jo and I sat between Mum and Dad reading *The Hobbit*, our two golden heads locked in an epic struggle for attention and the best princess dress. We have grown up, and the centrifugal force between parent and child has weakened over time, replaced by the new bonds we have made as we have created our own grown-up lives, our own families, our own security.

But though they are looser now, the older bonds remain. I felt them as I sat with Jo on the beach in Vietnam, I feel them as we four Grosses sit together in my parents' garden now. Layer on layer of experiences that only we share; our family shorthand, unique to us as it is to any family. We speak of *ice-creaming* things, in celebration of Jo's ability to hold on to a sweet treat for eons after I had finished. Jo and I pronounce our surname to rhyme with 'cross'. Of course we do – it was the only way to get around playground taunts, whereas Mum and Dad are happy to be Grosses, in the true American sense of the word. Only we can list our family pets in the correct chronological order. Bowie, the crazy desert dog who tore up the plastic grass in Mum's garden in Dubai, and his sidekick Useless Eustace, our grumpy kitten. Basil, the wise black Labrador whose soft ears provided consolation during my teenage heartbreaks, forever tormented by our farmyard cats Ratbag and Perfect Paws (can you guess which was mine and which was Jo's?). Sam and Lola, puppies born as I emerged from my cocoon, their hot Labrador bodies sleeping all day in the shade outside our house in France. All these creatures, the perfect furry backdrop to our four-square. (Surely Conan Doyle was right: 'A dog reflects the family life. Whoever saw a frisky dog in a gloomy family, or a sad dog in a happy one?') We share memories of places: rooms, homes, treehouses that my dad, thwarted architect that he is, has built for us. Even our tastebuds are formed by our inheritance, shaped by early exposure to mangoes, curry and Baskin-Robbins ice cream.

It is easy for me to forget all this as I focus my primal energies on the incipient destruction of my own First Family. But there are a mother and a father losing their girl, too, and a sister who never asked to be an only child. I am ashamed to say that their experience and the loss they will feel remain at the back of my mind, submerged under the blanket of emotion I have for my own children and Billy. I let the four-square make everything all right for me, just as they always have. But most of the time, I don't allow myself to imagine what this is like for them.

I am told that when we were young, Jo and I fought viciously. Naturally, I resented this little blonde thing who had stolen my prized place on Mummy's lap. Who was this interloper who pooed in the bath and laughed in my face when I professed disgust at her infantile ways? (I showed my anger by pushing her head underwater towards the offending object. Mum smacked my bottom, and I nursed my disgruntlement long enough for this to become a seminal event in my childhood.) The jigsaw puzzle I was given to 'celebrate' Jo's birth couldn't begin to compensate for her displacing me at the centre of my parents' universe. A few months in, I asked my mum anxiously, 'Is she staying?' Incomprehensibly, the answer seemed to be yes.

And so there we were, two little girls locked in a titanic battle. We were forced to share everything, from My Little Pony's Dream Castle to Mum's lap. And because there were two of us, and because we were both girls, we were (and we are) defined in relation to one another. We do it to ourselves, and our parents, teachers and friends do it to us. I was the tyrannical older sister, she was the victim. She was the patient to my doctor, the air hostess on our pretend plane, the serf to my princess. Eventually, Jo learned ways to subvert her bossy older sister. She taunted me till I walloped her, and then played the injured party to Mum. We would sit next to one another sweating through long car journeys, and she would pinch me surreptitiously until my patience snapped. As teenagers, I knew she was wearing something precious of mine when she dashed out of the house with a heavy coat and no backward glance. We once came to blows over a bottle of shampoo.

I say I am told about some of this, because despite the fighting, sibling loathing is not how I remember things. I may have ruled Jo's world with an iron grip, but once she escaped my dictatorial clutches she got her own back. While I was being a fat, nerdy little grub, she was tall, hot and effortlessly part of the Cooliverse. Now I am a bastion of the establishment, and she is the reflective, creative one. I make lists; she makes art. I buy high street; she buys vintage. Neither of us has our real hair colour any more, but when we did she was the real blonde and I was the mouse. Looking back, all of the pinching, tears and curses blur – what remains in focus is our mutual enmity towards our parents, and our closeness. We are protective of one another; I am red in tooth and claw when it comes to Jo. She brings out a fierceness in me matched only by what I feel for my children. When I was mid-finals (and going quite loopy) she came to my revolting student house, cooked me dinner, and then curled up in bed next to me. I always sleep soundly in a room with Jo. The noise of her breathing takes me back to the bedroom we once shared, with its Laura Ashley rose-printed duvets, and the dolls' house Dad made.

One of the reasons I elect to return to the beastly chemo ward time and time again is because I want to live to see Jo's children. They are, for the moment, a gleam in her eye. But I imagine a baby niece who like her mother will let loose little turds in the bath, horrifying her big-boy cousins. I long to feel another Gross baby bounce on my knee, to see our DNA reproduce itself. I want a little niece with her mother's blonde hair and blue eyes to hold my hand as we tour my beloved Museum of Costume in Bath, to jump with delight as I bring her handmade calico sundresses in bright West African prints. My skills as an aunt are unproven, but (I feel sure) exemplary.

What will life be like for Jo when she is left without her strait-laced elder sister? Does she become the *everywoman* daughter to fill the space I leave in the Gross four-square? I hope she doesn't have to take on all my seriousness and list-making alongside her creativity and gentleness. She is enough as she is. But if I were Jo, I would wish I had a spare sibling to fall back on. Emily Dickinson said she 'would like more sisters, that the taking out of one might not leave such stillness'. I can understand that. Where will she get her hand-me-downs from? Who will take over my role nagging her to stop smoking?

And then there is the four-square, which needs two sisters as it needs two parents: there are four chairs around our kitchen table, two ancient and battered Christmas stockings, two Father's Day cards on the mantelpiece. There should be two of us to balance the two of them, to bemoan their failing memories as we once winced at their musical tastes and Mum's penchant for pink leather. The balance of the four-square will be gone when I go. The remaining three will have to refashion themselves from square into triangle.

I can't shake this feeling that I am letting them all down. Wiping my parents' decrepit bottoms in twenty years' time was supposed to be *my job*, just as it is to wipe the peachy behinds of my offspring right now. That's not the end of it. I've always brought home good news: good exam results, sensible job, beautiful children and even (eventually) a respectable husband. I've laid all these life trophies down before my darling parents, anxious to please because that is how I show my love for them. I've never knowingly failed at anything in my life, and now I seem to be failing at hanging on to it. Their golden girl – the one who lives to please – may be gilded on the outside, but inside she is rotten. Dammit, I feel guilty.

Mum told me, after the operations and the recurrence, that she had come to see me like her favourite cardigan. It developed a hole that could be mended. Just moths having a nibble. But then she found another hole. And another. And it couldn't be mended any more. She tells me that losing me will be like losing a dear friend whose company you cherish. She says it is not the same as losing a young child. Her visceral, maternal urge to protect me, she says, has been transferred to my children. I get this; our relationship has changed over the years. I am no revolutionary. Not for me the rejection of parents' lifestyle and social mores. Instead I want to be friends with them, and I covet what they have. I envy their smart kitchen. Mum and I share poetry and shift dresses. Dad and I talk business and gardening. We argue over politics, though only to the extent of how far we are along the centre-left spectrum. They are friends and ideological fellow-travellers as well as parents.

When Mum says that losing me now is not the same as losing a dependent child, it comforts me. I can't carry anyone else's grief. But I wonder if it's true, or if she is, as ever, protecting me. I wonder because, despite my myopia, I have had a glimpse of my parents' reality. I've spent a lot of time in hospital, and during one of these sojourns – after my liver operation – there was a moment when everything about parental love was suddenly clear to me. Billy had brought the boys to the hospital to have an ice cream with me after tea, and he brought my mum too. I hadn't seen the kids since I'd been admitted to A&E the night before. I rushed up to give the sweaty, slightly odorous boys a hug. Obviously they resisted my cuddles, and I was left to ruffle their tousled heads while they told me purposefully about snakes and a fight with Fletcher. Mum hugged my arm while I was mid hair-ruffle. For an instant I viewed my life from outside, as if it were a home movie. Mum looked at me the way I look at them.

I saw then so clearly that my parents have the same treasure house of love for me as I have for my boys. But really, I already knew this. I had started to understand it when I hatched out of the grub stage. Slowly, over my twenties my parents became people, as well as providers of cash subsidies and free meals. They came into focus as formed human beings, with actual features and personalities. Then I had my own children, and suddenly I saw them sharply. Could anyone love anything as much as I loved my babies?

Aha. *That* is how they love me. Seeing with this clarity is painful, too. It makes me realise how completely, unspeakably crap it must be for them to watch me exist through this Nuisance. I know they would take my place in an instant. Yes, losing an adult daughter is like losing a best friend, but they will also mourn the little girl who curled up on their lap and cried, 'Lookatabook, shawee?' I am an adult, and their friend. But to them I am always their child, always one corner of the original four-square.

When I permit myself to think about this, I feel boundlessly lucky that I am the sick one, not either of my children. The other day, Mum reminded me of the story of the Greek harvest goddess Demeter and her daughter Persephone. Persephone – perhaps the original golden girl – was spotted by Hades, the lord of the underworld. He wanted her for his own, and stole her away to his land of the dead, leaving her heartbroken mother to search for her all across the land. Eventually, Demeter begged Persephone's father Zeus for help, and Zeus granted that she could be released from the underworld, provided she hadn't eaten or drunk anything in that dark subterranean place. Now, poor Persephone *had* eaten a few pome-granate seeds, so Zeus decreed that she could only spend half the year in the sunlit uplands of our world, and the remaining half-year amongst the shades of Hades. So Persephone and her mother have six months dancing in the sunshine, but every time Persephone returns to the underworld, Demeter is destroyed by loss all over again.

If either of my children died, my grief and anger would tear up the world like Demeter's did. I would claw at the earth of their graves. I would break up the sky and curse the soil so that nothing good could ever come of it again. I would be consumed by bitterness. None of the quiet, the strange content-ment I have now – no, rage and fury would rule. I read books like *Wave*, the memoir of Sonali Deraniyagala, who lost her husband and her two sons (and both her parents) in the tsunami of 2004, to take myself to the edge of grief and back again. When I return, I am grateful that it is me who is dying, not them. And I feel my parents' pain.

Billy had a conversation with his dad about this parental love thing. Billy's wise old dad said to him that a parent's love is like a ball. It gets passed on to each generation. But the ball only goes one way – from parent to child, and on to that child's children in turn. You don't expect to have the ball passed back to you by your own kids. Yes, of course we love our parents. We need them (however old we get, we always need them). But it is just a different kind of love from the sort you give a child. And as parents our job is to pass the ball forward, not to hang around waiting to get it back in the same form. We are our children's custodians, but they are not our possessions. In the words of Khalil Gibran, 'You may house their bodies but not their souls, For their souls dwell in the house of tomorrow, which you cannot visit.' We have to let our children find the world for themselves, without expecting heartfelt thank-yous for our efforts.

This realisation comforts me. It comforts me because I have never said the thanks I should have to my parents. But then again, even if I had lasted another fifty years, I wouldn't get – or expect – any thanks from my own children for my efforts. What goes around comes around, in the perfect symmetry of life. This comforts me, because in all the child-hood memories that I have, there is a notable absence. It is my parents, and specifically my mother. My early memories are those of a self-centred child, secure in her solipsism. I am the star, and my supporting cast is my peers, children of all ages (including the long-suffering Jo). My mum's Eighties perm and brightly coloured boilersuits don't really feature in my mental tableaux. Not because she wasn't there. Not because she didn't love me. No, quite the opposite: because she gave me love beyond compare, because she was always there, her presence is a given. She is the stage hand, pulling the strings behind my performance, the wardrobe mistress ensuring that my outfit is flawless, the prompter waiting just offstage should I falter with my lines. Her invisibility is a mark of the security she provided me. Had it been otherwise, she would feature more heavily, I have no doubt. So while I want my boys to remember every detail of me – of course I do, I'm still the star of the Kate show – if I really think about it, I would be content to be just a blur of blonde hair and a soft lap in their memories. That would be proof enough that I had done my job, as my mum did hers.

So, perhaps I alight on the truth about losing an adult child, even if it is more difficult to bear than what Mum and Dad will tell me. My parents will mourn Kate, always their daughter, now also their friend. But I won't see this from them, because they are passing the ball forward, looking after me every step of the way, just as they always have done. Of course they will have their own, distinct grief. But they will keep it to themselves. They know this story isn't about them. So they are there in the background, making things good. Encouraging me when I need courage. Reading to my children when I am too tired and broken to do it. Leaving food in my freezer, mowing the lawn, replacing the lightbulbs, quietly making every little thing all right.

6

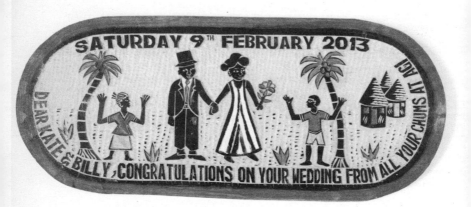

The Woman in the Arena

No man is an island entire of itself; every man is a piece of the continent, a part of the main; if a clod be washed away by the sea, Europe is the less, as well as if a promontory were, as well as any manner of thy friends or of thine own were; any man's death diminishes me, because I am involved in mankind. And therefore never send to know for whom the bell tolls; it tolls for thee.

JOHN DONNE, 'MEDITATIONS'

I have spent my short working life trying to save the world, one paperclip at a time. My bureaucrat heart beats strong, and it beats because I believe that the way a country is governed changes people's lives – for better or for worse. I have wanted to set my paper-clips down on the side of making things better, because I am – we all are – involved with mankind. We are part of the same enmeshed, complex web we call humanity, society, or simply *life*. We are tied by threads of compassion for one another, for people we know and people we will never meet. But these threads are fragile. We spin our ties like little spiders, and if we choose to stop spinning, our connection to the web – and the web itself – weakens and breaks.

How I ended up spending my working life in this way is really a series of fortuitous accidents. As Steve Jobs said, the difficult thing about careers is that you can't connect up the dots of your future in advance, only with the benefit of hindsight. My selection of dots – part choice, part chance, part a product of that mental landscape created in my early years – led me to a career in public service. But if I have learned anything in my working life, it's that virtues and vices are not conferred on you by your job title. The dots that really matter aren't the ones where you decide what you want to *do*, but how you want to *be*.

I spent my early years confidently expecting to become poet laureate (remember the extensive juvenilia?). I visited Westminster Abbey, aged about ten, to see the tombs in Poets' Corner, and marked out my final resting place somewhere between Chaucer and Tennyson. But there was something else going on behind this ambitious plan for a literary future. It began, I think, with Oscar Wilde's story 'The Young King'. There is, in this story, a young king in a land far away. This metrosexual little royal is a fan of luxury goods. For his coronation he has chosen to wear a 'robe of tissued gold', a 'ruby-studded crown', and a 'sceptre with rows and rings of pearls'. But on the eve of the ceremony he sees in a dream the terrible stories of how his rich garments were created. The sweatshop where his golden robe was woven. The little slave boy who died deep-sea diving for his pearls. The blood shed to mine the rubies on his crown.

Something about the story of this little lord stuck with me, buried underneath layers of wannabe Plath for years and years. The juvenilia was boxed up, and I fell into the bookworm's trap of sounding like someone else every time I tried to write. One day I was F. Scott Fitzgerald, with stories of teenage flappers (always getting pregnant, perhaps a reflection of the dire warnings from my form teacher given while rolling a condom onto a banana). Another, my voice would be Holden Caulfield's and the world full of phoneys. I over-identified with Toni Morrison and the school of African-American women writers. Of course I did: the experience of slavery, of black womanhood, of oppression – all that spoke *so* strongly to my over-privileged fourteen-year-old self. The more I read, the more other voices filled my head. I stopped writing, and instead started wondering how I could earn a living in the most glamorous fashion possible.

I spent my undergraduate years hoping to get into advertising, largely on the basis that I believed it to be full of hot young things who lounged on beanbags in their glamorous Soho offices. But somewhere along the way to real life, Mum suggested that the civil service might be an option. I don't quite know how she knew it would suit me, given that her main interaction with that world had been through

Yes, Minister. Once I'd been offered it, actually taking my first job in government was a rare triumph of my better nature. I compared the dark, fortress-like walls of the Home Office, replete with endless boxy offices, stuffed with papers and middle-aged men with dandruff, with the glossy life I could have in Soho, and the grub wanted glamour. But there was something about what the dandruffy men were working on which hooked me. Intractable problems. Impossible choices where there was no right or wrong, but a decision still had to be taken. How to punish the boy who stole my mobile phone on Clapham Common, for example. Dole out some rough justice and rip off his thin little teenage arm? (To my eternal discredit I did my best on that front, sustaining a broken hand in my struggle to retain my treasured Nokia brick.) Lock him up? Or try to understand that he was only sixteen, hadn't had the advantages I'd enjoyed, and deserved a chance to get some qualifications and make a go of things?

The idea that there wasn't actually just black and white, but rather infinite shades of grey, was energising in a way I hadn't anticipated. I liked the fact that while the commentators could comment and the complainers complain, secure up there on the moral high ground, ultimately someone had to decide. The young king and his rubies, long buried somewhere in my hinterland, were re-emerging.

So I stumbled into this world of government, where my job was to balance the arguments, to work out what was possible, and to give choices to the people the voters had chosen to make decisions. That is democracy, and that is politics. That is Theodore Roosevelt's 'man in the arena', with his – or her – face covered with dust and sweat and blood (as she meticulously affixes paperclips to files and provides evidence-based, politically neutral advice). Because, in Roosevelt's words, 'It is not the critic who counts; not the man who points out how the strong man stumbles, or where the doer of deeds could have done them better.'

Sometimes the world seems full of people who are happiest carping from the sidelines, desperate for the merry-go-round of modernity to stop so they can get off and retreat to an imagined golden age. In *The Lord of the Rings*, Frodo wishes he could stop the ride and not take up the awful mantle of ring-bearer. 'I wish it need not have happened in my time,' he says. Gandalf answers, 'So do I ... and so do all those who live to see such times.' I feel Frodo's pain. But the people I admired have always been those who dared to get off the fence, because if you stay on it, nothing ever happens. Those who seek out complexity and messiness over neatness and order. Those who say, 'This is what I believe in, so judge me for it.' Those who look at the world as if it were a fairground, and say, 'Give me a ride and take me to the future, whatever it brings.' (Perhaps this explains my heroine-worship of Elizabeth I and Queen Victoria, two women who seemed pretty happy in the arena.)

If, like me, you are the kind of person who wants to stand in the arena, then there is really only one place you aspire to work. The heart of it all – the centre of the centre: the White House, the Elysée Palace, where the kitchen cabinet meets, the inner sanctum. In my case, the black door to No. 10 Downing Street held a fascination for me from the moment I first saw it, later on the same day on which I'd marked out my future spot in Poets' Corner. That door oozed power, and I desperately wanted to know what went on behind it (because, you see, it is possible to be involved in mankind and also to be a deeply ambitious young lady). By a series of haphazard choices and lucky accidents, fifteen years after I first saw that black door I ended up working behind it.

It was all I had expected, yet somehow less. For starters, the 'smart' part of Downing Street is decorated rather like a posh country hotel – a little bit chintzy, comforting, rather old-fashioned. Belowstairs is different – a warren of poky, nondescript offices which encircle the epicentre of power, the prime minister's study. When the boss is in the office, the whole place hums. When he's out in his constituency or away at a summit, it is quiet: a Trusthouse Forte hotel in the off-season, slightly past its best and smelling faintly of damp. But even then – especially then – the past provides an edge. There are ghosts around every corner. On those quiet days I would stand in the Cabinet Room, looking out onto Horse Guards Parade, and think of the oil lamps Earl Grey feared in 1914 would not be lit again in his lifetime. I would walk up the great staircase lined with pictures of former prime ministers, and test myself on their stories. Which one was murdered in office? Which one was a byword for nepotism, the inspiration for the phrase 'Bob's your uncle'?* After meetings in Lady Thatcher's erstwhile study, I took particular joy in using her avocado-coloured lavatory.

I was called a private secretary. I wouldn't blame you for assuming that meant I was a typist who provided extras on the side. But the job of a private secretary is, for the bureaucrat, a respectable and coveted one. There is the elected politician, and then there is his or her Person. Their second brain, gate-keeper, protector, adviser, bag-carrier, head of random tasks – from the sublime (decision-making, speech-writing, fact-finding, crisis-alleviating) to the ridiculous (down-calming, morale-boosting, make-up-checking). My job, back then, required preparing the prime minister for everything he said in Parliament. Every utterance of policy on every situation was my responsibility (well, it was his. But it

---

* For readers without *The Pedant's Guide to 10 Downing Street* at hand, the answers are: (1) Spencer Perceval; (2) Lord Salisbury, uncle of Arthur Balfour.

was my job to ferret out the facts of the matter so he could work out what he wanted to say). Plus, I advised the prime minister on a selection of the aforementioned fat, juicy, intractable problems. On my list were home affairs (whether or not to let foreigners into the country, how to punish my mobile-phone thief), terrorism, hunting with dogs (really, this was a big issue. I can hardly credit it these days, but it was), food and farming (whether or not to kill the badgers responsible for spreading TB in cows, quarantining parrots with avian flu), and a ragbag of other things, usually to do with politicians being flayed by the media at the height of a scandal (sex, money, otherwise), or constitutional affairs, which I'm afraid I considered a tedious policy layby (I would rather raze the House of Lords to the ground than spend another moment of my life debating how it should be reformed).

The responsibility of all this sat well with me, so long as I remembered Oscar Wilde's young king and his luxury goods. The choices made by those in power are never without repercussions. People are not statistics, and behind every decision to stop migrants from entering the country or to take a different approach to supporting difficult children at school there are lives changed, families made and broken, misery and joy. And I had to remember that although I spoke for power, I didn't have power myself. Sometimes it was easy to get confused, and for the audacity of being so young and being behind that black door to turn to arrogance.

It is one thing to understand and feel responsibility for what happens to people who live on the streets of our cities. That is mind-blowing enough. But our compassion has to stretch to those we will never meet, those who live far away, whose lives will never touch ours directly, but to whom we are connected in this fragile web. The young king's territory was borderless, and so is ours. And really, in our little lives right now we are inexplicably and incredibly blessed. I grew up in a time of peace and relative plenty, and to me that feels like the norm. But I don't have to do a long sweep of history, or look very far afield, to realise what a gilded aberration I have existed in. Most people, in most of the world, are engaged in something which more closely resembles a medieval – or at least industrial-age – battle for survival, for security, for the prosperity and comfort we in this country take for granted. Most children don't have the chances mine were born with. Most women wouldn't have made it to the high-tech operating table I was lifted onto on that day of my first diagnosis, let alone had all the brilliant medical care I've had since then.

So, although I spent the early bit of my working life wrestling with the problems of this country, it has always been the big world that animates me. After four years I left No. 10 and moved to Cambridge, and there I found my golden ticket: an invitation to do a job which would change things for me just as much as those early encounters with the mongoose and the Nepalese Living Goddess. Tony Blair had decided he wanted to spend a portion of his post-prime ministerial life working in Africa. There he'd met leaders he respected, and had watched them struggle to govern countries broken by civil war, genocide and famine, with none of the systems of state we in the UK have built up over hundreds of years of bureaucratic structures which translate money and ideas into reality. As Ellen Johnson Sirleaf, president of Liberia, put it:

> There you stand, trying to rebuild a nation in an environment of raised expectations and short patience ... After all, they voted for you because they had confidence in your ability to deliver – immediately. Only you cannot. Not because of the lack of financial resources, but simply because the capacity to implement whatever change you have in mind does not exist.

One country above all others changed the way I thought about my career. Look across Africa, from west to east, from bolshie little Liberia to massive, exuberant Kenya. Settle your gaze on a landscape of lakes and volcanoes, bang-splat in the middle of the continent. Here, in 1994, over the course of a hundred days, nearly a million people were killed. 'Decimation,' wrote Philip Gourevitch, 'means the killing of every tenth person in a population, and in the spring and summer of 1994 a programme of massacres decimated the Republic of Rwanda.'

Nearly a million people murdered by their friends, neighbours and colleagues. A generation destroyed, or carrying the weight of the destruction they had caused. The state had engineered a genocide, and in its wake the state combusted. What happened next? The Rwandan people voted, but as well as choosing their government they wanted to know they could sleep safe in their beds. Government must deliver security before anything else. Once a mother knows the family she has created will not be ripped apart before her eyes, she starts to ask questions about clean water for her children to drink, bed-nets to keep them safe from malarial mosquitoes, roads to take the mangoes she has grown to market, and electricity so she can study at night for a better job.

These things, which we take for granted, do not happen by magic. They require the state to act. Decisions, money, and after that, the steady drip-drip of bureaucracy to make sure the decisions are followed up and the money is well spent. Meetings. Coordination. Updates. More decisions. Paperclips. When I first visited Rwanda, thirteen years after the genocide, I found a cadre of public servants committed to refashioning their country. But they were young (even by my standards), and for some of them this was their first job since leaving a refugee camp. Switching on a computer and typing memos was, understandably, not part of their skill-set. But it was part of mine, it was in my bureaucrat's blood. At the same time, I knew that the job of the man (or woman) at the top is a lonely one, and that the only person who really understands what it feels like to bear the responsibility of leading a country is someone who has, well, led a country. Rwanda showed me that there was the germ of an idea here, an idea that made my bureaucrat heart beat faster.

Today, seven years after I stepped off the plane in Kigali, there exists an organisation called the Africa Governance Initiative. I was its founding chief executive. Tony Blair is its patron. As I write, there are more than fifty passionate, committed and brilliant people working across nine countries for this little organisation with a big idea: that government has to work better for the poorest people in the world.

*   *   *

When I was working in Africa, I didn't need to remind myself about the young king. People's stories were up close and personal. Geoffrey, the student I met at the National University of Rwanda who told me how he hid in the forest for months after his family were killed in the genocide, how he emerged and was sponsored through school by a kindly foreigner, about his dreams for the future and for his hilly, beautiful country. Kadie, who helped our very first team get themselves settled in Sierra Leone, showing us what to buy in the market and how to get the air conditioning fixed, who died when she was younger than I am, leaving a seven-year-old son behind – and how this wasn't unusual in a country where you are beating the odds if you reach your fifties. Albert, our driver in Liberia, who called me 'Bosslady' and who had lived through civil war, with all its mutilation of limbs, child soldiers and endless fighting for control of those accursed, sparkly rocks. The people I met in Juba, the capital of South Sudan, Africa's newest country – a 'city' which viewed from the air was just a tiny tarmac crossroads, with dirt tracks spreading out like arteries into the wide-open spaces of a country the size of France. In the heart of that dusty place, the young woman who worked late into the night in the president's office, her own bureaucrat heart beating faster and faster as her newborn country fought for survival.

None of these stories is about politics, though it is worth saying that politics is not a dirty word as far as I am concerned. Politicians can be people of principle, just like the rest of us. Of course (*of course*) this is not universally the case; but I have learned much from the politicos I have observed. I have seen someone choose between their own political future and the right economic choice for their country, because few politicians can survive raising the price of rice in a starvation economy. I have watched someone maintain his humanity, generosity of spirit and optimism despite being torn down daily by thousands of people who sought nothing less than his personal destruction and humiliation. I have learned, by watching a leader institute a totally new justice system to try the perpetrators of genocide, that sometimes you have to discard convention, because the status quo would have taken a hundred years to deliver any sort of peace to the hundreds of thousands of accused and their victims.

Such stories are not about which party is in power; they are simply about people, who need to be able to rely on a system, on their state. I always understood this intellectually. But now that my own family is in trouble, I get it in a visceral, kick-in-the-stomach kind of way. The desire to protect your children, especially when your own future is uncertain. The need for financial security for your family. What it feels like to be dependent on people, to need so much from others when all you want is control of your life. How fear can shape a family and the decisions you take. I'm abundantly aware that hardship is a spectrum, of which I am at an exceptionally privileged, lucky and well-supported end. But I see the whole of that spectrum more clearly now. I see the suffering, and I am overwhelmed by what people will do out of compassion for others. Yes, the threads that bind us together are fragile, easily ruptured by ties to self, to tribe, to race, to friends, to family. But that they are there *at all* is a reason for unconquerable gladness.

There are stories, in Rwanda, of Hutus who instead of killing, protected the victims, paying with their own lives. Philip Gourevitch tells of an attack on a school. The killers told the children to split themselves into groups of Tutsis and Hutus. The children refused to do so even as the attackers opened fire, and died side by side, because they loved one another. These stories of compassion sustain hope when it seems there is nothing left to be hopeful about. They show me what it really means to be involved with mankind.

In a different way, so does what my mother and sister have chosen to do with their working lives. If I have been drawn to the intellectual space where bad and good decisions are made, they have been drawn to immediate, real intervention in children's lives. I remember Mum coming home from her job as an educational psychologist with a black eye because she had been headbutted by one of the boys she had been supporting. This shocked us at home, and made me wonder why she was trying to help these terribly disturbed children when they were so utterly ungrateful. Likewise little sister Jo, surrounded all week by thirty five-year-olds, half of whom didn't speak English when they turned up in her class, some of whom were angry and violent, others hothoused by overbearing parents who had taught them to read and count, but not to play. Mum and Jo have never needed to remind themselves of the story of the young king, because they spend their lives with the pearl divers – and that, of course, is far harder than sitting in an office pontificating about paperclips.

I don't want you to come away with the impression that I believe public service is the only vocation that matters, or in fact the only way to be involved with mankind. Nor should you be under the misapprehension that I am a self-sacrificing angel who will give up anything to help others. (Oh no. I am ambitious and driven, and want to succeed as much as the next woman – probably more, if I'm honest.) The last thing I want is for my children to read this and feel as though only one life choice would have pleased me. That is nonsense. Job titles are irrelevant ciphers, not the truth about who we are. There is an intrinsic value in being a bin man as much as an astrophysicist, an artist or a nurse, an investment banker or a teacher. What counts is not just what you do, but *how* you do it.

It's down to choices. More of Gandalf's wisdom: 'All we have to decide is what to do with the time that is given to us.' Most of those choices come down to whether or not you treat other people with compassion. In the first instance, the people directly around you. We are all like icebergs, presenting only a small part of ourselves for view. Underneath the water is a dense mass, so dense that sometimes even we ourselves can't see most of it. We can choose what we reveal of ourselves, but we can also choose how much we want to see of other people. The more you show, the more you seek, the more involved you are with mankind. Then there are the people at one remove, all of those who will end up being affected by the law you write or the tree you grow or the product you sell. Under the law of the butterfly flapping its wings, of course, you won't always be able to make everyone's lives better. You will end up unknowingly doing things wrong, hurting people; I am sure I have left my fair share of collateral damage along the way, wittingly and otherwise. But you can do your best to behave in a way that is thoughtful of a world bigger than yourself. You can be responsible in how you do things, remembering that you are blessed with the gorgeousness of free will.

Compassion is often seen as the province only of the religious. It shouldn't be. It is for all of us. But I have to admit that though it animates my life, I still find that simple truth hard to live by. My little world is ordered, and I like to *choose* when my munificence will be offered. The other day I woke to hear an old, drunk, very distressed man falling down around the bins outside our house. I didn't go out to help, but I heard my neighbours do so. I was at church recently, having a nice quiet think and feeling very pleased with myself for finding some inner peace, and I was nothing but angry when a homeless guy came in and started disturbing things for me. I am Eliot's Chorus, watching Thomas Becket's downfall and begging not to be involved. I am the UN official who heard news of mass murder in Rwanda but was too nervous to call it genocide.

Despite my weakness, I am involved. I know that it isn't enough to be big-hearted only on the days I choose – when I'm at work and *doing good* with my paperclips, but not when I'm in the sanctity of my own home or doing something I consider precious *for me*. Compassion has to be practised – maybe a bit like yoga, but without the heavy breathing – if it is to become a habit. But, like yoga, I struggle with this. It doesn't come easy, though being shocked out of my gilded cage by the Nuisance has made me try harder and love more than ever I did before. But as my time ebbs away, I find I turn in on myself and my own family's struggle. Then I try to remind myself of that mad genius William Blake's words:

> We are put on earth for a little space,
> that we might learn to bear the beams of love.

7

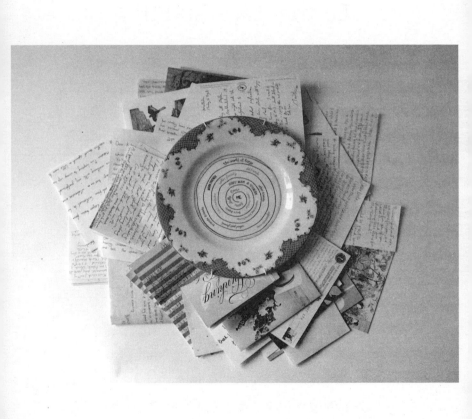

Earthquakes, and the Light They Let In

There is only one way to defeat the sorrow and sadness of life – with laughter and rejoicing. Bring out your good dishes, put on your good clothes, no sense hoarding them ... bring them all out, Roxana, and enjoy them.

ROHINTON MISTRY, *FAMILY MATTERS*

I would do anything not to be writing this book. But I am, and though it fills me with rage that I won't be there to watch my boys grow into men, there is a strange gladness to my heart. The time I have had since I became ill has been beyond precious; this strange, razor-like clarity is something I wouldn't have found had the worst not happened. Nor would

I have found my voice, the time to tell this story, or what really matters in this magnificent life. Really, it's no silver lining. Hell no. But if the suffering my children will experience at too early an age transmutes them, in just a tiny way, then they will be happier and even more remarkable people because of it. Of course, this is not a bargain I want to make. No amount of lucid self-knowledge is recompense for what my family will lose. But perhaps, just perhaps, where I am because of all this will change you too, and that matters. So, we have to talk about suffering, pain, about not getting what you want or what you deserve. Because an earthquake will hit everyone's life at some point, and I have something to say about how it feels, and how the people around you can respond.

Though my life has, until now, been gilded and lovely, that is not the case for most people, most of the time, in most of the world. Nothing can protect us from harm. The universe is a random, arbitrary place. If there is a God, he sure isn't an interventionist who will cradle you in security all your life. He's as much in control as we are – not a bloody lot.

Billy is a great lover of Boethius, and I see him reading *The Consolations of Philosophy* before we see the doctors for the latest news on my cancerous progress, reminding himself of Lady Fortune's words that 'Inconsistency is my very essence; it is the game I never cease to play as I turn my wheel in its ever changing circle … as I bring the top to the bottom and the bottom to the top.' I have had days, since my diagnosis, when I felt myself at the bottom of the wheel; and in my heart of hearts I know there will be far worse to come for me and for those I love. With each birthday the boys will understand a little more what they have lost. Billy has half a lifetime ahead of him without me. I don't know what other sorts of pain my family will come up against later in their lives. But I do know that trying to predict that future is like trying to catch a jellyfish. Too slippery. Painful. Totally pointless. The fact is, whether you come to it from a Christian perspective – or indeed from most of the other faiths – or if, like Billy, you believe in none of the above, there is really no accounting for the random good and bad luck of the world. Realising that life isn't an arc which soars ever upwards providing you pay your dues and behave well is actually quite a release. Because then you can get on with the business of dealing with what you have, of finding meaning in suffering, and of seeing joy in the everyday.

People approach me with trepidation nowadays. I suspect they stand outside our front door working out how to compose themselves, wondering how bad I will look, if this is the last time we'll see each other, what on earth to say. Most of the time I disappoint on all counts: my happiness, my good humour and my 'bonny' radiance come as a surprise. But to explain why it is possible to be happy when you are – objectively speaking – at the bottom of Lady Fortune's wheel, I first need to answer the other gnawing question people have in their heads when they see me. How does it feel to be told you are going to die?

There is a raw agony that comes when the earthquake first hits. When we were told that I had cancer, and then again when we were told it had come back, and that this time there wasn't a hope of a cure. The agony will return when we are told I have weeks left, not months. I can feel it threatening even as I write, with my treatment options running out. That initial period after impact is searing. Now, I look back on the days we've had following Bad News, and I can remember almost every instant, in that way you do after the big events of your life. What I did. What I said to whom. The words that kept going round in my head: Not Yet, Not Yet. How I kept expecting the oncologist to tell me that my scans had 'lit up like a Christmas tree', because it was December, because we had just decorated our tree, and because that is what I had read someone say in a book. How the image I had in my head of death was of me in the back of a black taxi, leaving an awesome party before the end, just when everyone else was starting to have real fun. I remember Billy crying and telling me his heart was broken. I remember asking the best woman and Mum if the boys would be all right, seeking assurance that these surrogate mother figures would do what was needed. I remember what Oscar and Isaac said when I told them my tummy hurt was back, and I had to start having my sleepy medicine again, and how they reacted with absolute horror that we couldn't go swimming together any more. This, truly, was the end of their little world.

There was a weight of misery which went to bed with me at night, which I woke up with in the morning, and which I lugged around all day. I sometimes disposed of it briefly, because making banana muffins is a brilliant distraction. But it was there, all the time, and tears were quick to come. When I tell you what happened next, remember that I am not unusually unfeeling, but am basically wired for happiness. The sadness left me. Or perhaps it is fairer to say it settled in, it became part of my mental furniture, rather than a monster which inhabited my mind against my will. The sadness and I came to an accommodation with one another: if I let it out for a good wail every few days, it wouldn't assail me at inopportune moments. It would leave me space for other things. For me, at least, the acute period of misery after impact was short-lived – days or weeks. I think this was because we humans cannot exist in a state of heightened emotion for long. We are programmed to normalise, and that is what happens, even after the worst news imaginable. The last few years have followed this pattern – punctuated by short periods of awfulness, and then a gradual levelling out as we found the ground beneath our feet. I can only hope that I will continue to find that sure ground as things get worse.

So, the earth finds its place again after the quake, and a new normal begins. What happens to sadness and fear then? They come and go. Most of the time they rest quietly inside you, no longer something that thumps you with a punch when you wake. Not a reason to be fearful in the night; more a reality which requires managing. In my case, dying has been no quick sprint, though the pace is picking up. Bearing all the medical interventions and the anxiety and the fear about the future is more like the lengthy runs Billy goes on. He tells me (since I'm not one to take on a marathon myself) that it's mile twenty-two or so which is worst. Sort of near the end, but not really that close, and anyway by then it's raining buckets and you're slogging up a hill. You get the analogy.

The tough bit is not the start, it's the bit where you just have to put your head down and keep going; it's an endurance sport. Living with the after-effects of the quake is much harder than surviving the initial impact. There is a point when everyone else has gone back to normal life, when the spotlight isn't on you and your crisis any more, and it is then that things are at their toughest.

There is a third state, between crisis and endurance: uncertainty. Living with this is my Achilles heel. I am a woman to whom control is everything – see how I am trying to control the world even now, by fixing it in print for perpetuity? But I cannot control *this*, I can't game the outcome, I can't decide how the cancer inside me grows, how quickly, where it attacks next, whether or for how long my drugs do the business, how much pain I am in.

I am not used to this uncertain terrain. In every other aspect of my life, diligence and hard work have been rewarded with my getting what I want. I am a competent sort of person, passing my exams, getting stuff done at work, somehow even scraping through my driving test first time. I'm a golden girl, a people-pleaser, someone who is used to graft and a pleasant smile being rewarded. Yes, the world I lived in was uncontrollable. I couldn't prevent the suicide bombs that hit London on 7 July 2005, and nothing I could do would stop over two hundred Nigerian school-girls from being abducted by fanatics, or the world's newest country from tearing itself apart in civil war. But somehow all that was all right, because if I worked hard enough I believed I could nudge things, just incrementally, in a way that helped. I have a foolish faith in my own impact, as you can see. And this *completely* unjustifiable confidence has stood me in good stead – up till now.

It is hard for anyone to be at the mercy of forces outside their control, but it is especially hard for a control freak. Uncertainty is debilitating, confi-dence-sapping, anger-inducing. An important piece of identity is surrendered. Of course, the sense of being in charge is always a thin veneer waiting to be cracked like ice on a pond. But having it wrenched away so completely has changed me. My unthink-ing, buoyant self-confidence in my ability to make things *just so* has gone. Now the endless possibility of doom creeps into my thoughts in a way it didn't before: if life can go so spectacularly wrong for us in one way, what's to stop further calamities? What if Billy is killed in a car crash? Or one of the surrogate mothers gets sick? There is no law to say we've had our fair share of strife, and nothing I can do will fix Afterwards to make it safe.

Over the past couple of years I have explored different routes to find a way to live with this uncertainty. Mind over matter, to begin with. Yoga. Meditation. Cognitive behavioural therapy. It helps, it really does (it's always a pleasant indulgence to explore the inner reaches of the self). But frankly all this quietude doesn't touch the sides of the gaping hole that cancer has blasted through my sense of assurance. I turned to the Raymond Carver poem 'What the Doctor Said' a lot, at the beginning of all this.

> He said it doesn't look good
> he said it looks bad in fact real bad
> he said I counted thirty-two of them on one lung
>   before

Earthquakes, and the Light They Let In

I quit counting them
I said I'm glad I wouldn't want to know
about any more being there than that
he said are you a religious man do you kneel down
in forest groves and let yourself ask for help
when you come to a waterfall
mist blowing against your face and arms
do you stop and ask for understanding at those
    moments
I said not yet but I intend to start today
he said I'm real sorry he said
I wish I had some other kind of news to give you
I said Amen and he said something else
I didn't catch and not knowing what else to do
and not wanting him to have to repeat it
and me to have to fully digest it
I just looked at him
for a minute and he looked back it was then
I jumped up and shook hands with this man who'd
    just given me
something no one else on earth had ever given me
I may have even thanked him habit being so strong

I have started kneeling down in forest glades and old, cold churches and asking for help. The God I find there – the one who helps me cling on to a still small voice of calm – is the God of churches at smokefall, a God who swims in cold seas, inhabits high mountains and wild places. Being outside, amongst nature, amongst all of this is the one unfailing way I have found to stop my Achilles heel from crippling me. I can see why uncertainty makes people give up. I can completely see it. Imagine wondering every day if your loved ones will survive the day, because you live in a war zone. Will they make it home from work or school, or will a bomb maim them? Will they get pulled over at a roadblock because of the tribe they come from or what they believe? Will they be shot by a sniper on the way home from market? Our family's little tragedy pales in comparison to this, and that is the other thing that I try to remind myself of in the forest glade.

So there it is, the earthquake and its aftermath, laid bare for you. Seeing all these miserable words compacted together on the page makes me feel rather desolate. But that is because I haven't left space between my sentences to let the light in. Of course, in real life we have let it stream onto us.

The thing about an earthquake is that it ripples out for miles, shaking the ground, causing buildings to collapse and fault-lines to open in unexpected places. If you are at the epicentre you are only concerned with your family's survival, fixing their injuries and shoring up your home. The basics come first. But as the tectonic plates move, those further out are affected too; rocked by aftershocks, worried about those they know at the heart of the quake, anxious about their own future, desperate to know what they can do to help. The story in this book is the story of those people, too, and what they have done for us. I hold it out to you because you will do the same for someone, someday.

What does *do the same* mean? As you read this, hold the image of the spiral on the plate at the beginning of this chapter in your head. Is it a snail, a yogic symbol, or a Richter-scale event? It doesn't much matter; I stole it from the *LA Times* while I was recuperating from my liver operation in the States, and you can interpret it as you will. It is the best picture of my world that I can give you, and I suspect you will find it applicable to almost any family crisis you find yourself involved in. In the centre is me, the person who is dying. In the next circle out is our little foursome of a family. Sort of in the same bracket, but sort of not, are our parents, brothers and sisters. Outside that, a handful of our dearest friends – godparents to our children, the best men and women. Outside that – and this is a big, blurry, happy set of categories – others whom I love, but who are one degree removed. Colleagues. Old friends from work, university or school. Aunts and uncles. Outside that, people I know, but who I'm not properly in touch with: former housemates, friends' other halves, my husband's colleagues, an old boss, ex-boyfriends, school-gate mums. And so on, until you get to the world at large.

The spiral has one simple rule: you provide support only to those closer to the centre than you. And you expect support from those further out than you. To put it bluntly, you can only emotionally dump on people in circles further out than your own. I can weep on anyone, but no one gets to weep on me. (Of course you're sad that I'm dying, but I just don't need to hear you snuffle snottily that you're so devastated that I'm going to leave my children motherless. Hold it together, go cry on someone else.) Don't assume that you should crowd towards the centre of the spiral. Leave us space to breathe. The shoulder to cry on, the bunch of flowers, the pre-cooked dinner might be even more helpful to someone else. My mum, who is your friend. My sister, who is your colleague. My best woman, who is the girl you played with at primary school and have loved ever since.

When it comes to the spiral, it is natural to gravitate towards the practicalities. To want to feed people, take the children out, give a lift to hospital appointments. We all want to feel we are *doing something*. But there is no blanket list to suit all families and all occasions, and you will have to work hard to establish a rhythm of assistance which supports but doesn't intrude. You should ask what we need, and if you are met with silence, make suggestions. And then ask again in six months' time, because the chances are that that is the point at which everyone else will have stopped offering help. And if you still don't get an answer? Well, maybe just do it. Managing all the help that is offered is tiring. Sometimes I just want someone to sweep in uninvited and quietly do the ironing, and not ask for any acknowledgement of the good deed they have done. Remember, this is not about *you*. The point is not to burnish your halo, but to help.

Those of us at the centre of the spiral need some room to exhale. But we also need to know that you are there. I grant that this is a fine line to tread. When we had the news that my cancer had returned, this time without hope of a cure, from some quarters there was silence. I understand that. If this were happening to someone else, I would have been one of the silent bystanders, sympathetic but convinced that whatever I said would be a blundering imposition, that it would make things worse to say the wrong thing than nothing at all. I would have been wrong. The *only* answer is to say something. There is really nothing you can say that will make things worse, after all. And we don't expect great words of wisdom or solace. I just want this shit to be acknowledged, to know that you are offering me reassuring hand-squeezes (whether virtual or actual).

Don't be afraid to visit. I know there will be a moment, as you stand outside the house, when you will wish you hadn't come, but really, it will be OK. I'm still me. You can tell me I look great, even if I don't. But please don't treat me as if I'm a dying saint who has granted you an audience in her final hours. Don't hold our moments together in some precious reverence. Don't make me feel as if this is the last time we will meet. The invalid craves normality, not exceptionalism.

I expected support, but not solace. But solace has come, from inner circles and from outer reaches of the spiral. After the initial silence, I have been amazed by people's ability to reach me with their words. I am touched by their ability to open themselves to me. 'Only connect,' as E.M. Forster said. The word has been hijacked by slick Americans talking about how to network at conferences ('Have you connected with Mark? He's doing amazing things with former child soldiers in the Central African Republic'). But at its root is the sharing of lives, sharing which builds friendships and communities. People open themselves up to me, revealing the pain of their own loss (mothers, fathers, friends, children), their loneliness, their fears. What has helped them through their own earthquakes, big and small. The story of my Palestinian friend's family, splintered across a Middle East which is fracturing over and over again as I write. The happiness he has found with a Jewish guy in New York, conflicting with his desire to be *at home* and making a difference in his own backyard. Not wanting to abandon his loved ones for an easy life. Choices and uncertainty as geopolitics as well as family politics. The story of a friend who has spent years exorcising her depressive demons, and who has found solace in writing. She has a heart as big as the African countries we worked in together, and she is willing to open it to the world. Someone's little brother (who will be forever a lanky child in my mind) telling me about his stillborn child with a dignity and peace he must have acquired somewhere between eleven and grown-up.

But I'm not just about the sad stories. Don't assume that I don't want to share your joy. I do, even more than before. My whiff of envy at a new house, a cash windfall, a delightful new baby, magically disappeared when my cancer arrived. Now I just need more good news in my life. I love to be told about an awesome new job. I long for news of pregnancies and births. And though I spend a lot of time navigating the big things in life, I've never been more interested in trivialities. Let us sit around the table with and bitch about horrible colleagues. Tell me about the embarrassing crop of old-lady hair that sprouts from your chin, untamed by the ladies who try to thread it away. Describe your children's latest irritating misdemeanours. If you are lucky, I will tell you about my trivialities too. How I hate to look at my fat round face in the mirror. How consumed I am by an obsession with Crunchie bars. How scared I am of the toad that lives in the back garden and jumps over my feet as I write in the sunshine.

There is something to be said about the *how* of saying all of this, as well as the *what*. The best communications are gentle, thoughtful, offering news and love, devoid of overwhelming suggestions or demands. I don't need to hear your theory about the latest cancer-busting injections of mistletoe, or that I should accept the eternal love of Jesus Christ as the only cure for my imminent death. And the best communications certainly don't require a reply. Can you imagine how soul-destroyingly dull it would be for me to spend all day telling people *how I am*? Yawn. I want to be communicated with. I love to be remembered in this strange house-arrest I sometimes feel I am under. But I dread the burden of reciprocation. I know this is not the polite way we normally do things, but I figure I can break the rules now; so make it all right, and sign off with a breezy 'No need to reply.'

The written word has a beauty of its own, so much more so than electronica. I love to be indulged with letters and cards, which can be read at leisure and treasured by my beloveds forever. I have boxes of letters received in the past few years. Behind those, there are boxes of the letters from before: cards from Billy, letters written to school friends, my stash of pre-Billy Darling letters, 'stiff in their cardboard coffins', as Carol Ann Duffy put it. Fragments of all my past lives stored up to gather dust and to remind people that once, I existed.

Sometimes I sit with these boxes of letters in front of me and let the papers spill out over my feet. All those words. Pictures. Memories. Love. The spiral holds me tightly and squeezes my hand. It whispers Julian of Norwich's calming mantra:

All shall be well, and all shall be well, and all manner of thing shall be well.

8

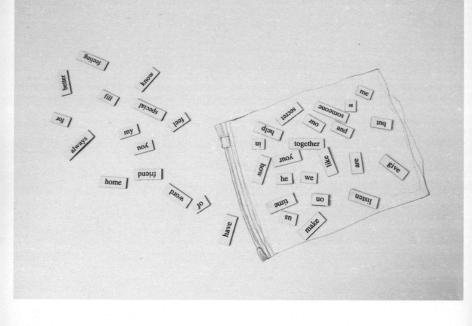

Cantus Firmus

What a man can be, he must be.

A.H. MASLOW, *A THEORY OF HUMAN MOTIVATION*

In another life, it is 2058, and I am eighty. I am sitting in a comfortable chair writing my memoirs. My paperclips are laid to one side, my dancing days are done. I am writing down the stories of the countries I have travelled to, places I have seen change before my eyes during a long career as an international stateswoman, a lady of influence, someone who has made the world around her a better place. In this ridiculously pleasing little reverie I am somewhere between Hillary Clinton, Angelina Jolie and Sheryl Sandberg. You see, I think I could have been a contender. For what, I don't quite know. Lacking any sense of a glass ceiling, and full of the confidence of youth, I thought I was going somewhere in the world. Not Hollywood, I grant you, or high political office, or the millionaires' club. But I was doing what I loved, and there was the promise of more of the same ahead. The Nuisance took that away. And though losing that imaginary professional future matters far, far less than losing a future with my children, still it leaves me wondering who I am without all that.

I've got history with this question of definition. It surfaced when I had the Knights. As the pioneering US feminist Charlotte Perkins Gilman said, 'It is not sufficient to be a mother; an oyster can be a mother.' Intellectually I agreed, but mummying filled me to the brim. How could I work by day when I spent my nights suckling twin boys? They had drunk me dry, metaphorically as well as literally. Their perfect four feet and rosebud lips had erased the memory of the woman who sat in the officials' box in the Houses of Parliament every Wednesday. I was no longer the bosslady to anyone at all. My previous selves dissolved in a lake of breast milk.

My disintegration should have been predictable. The idea of myself as a grown-up, professional woman was built on shaky ground, an edifice constructed of what I had done, not who I was. Each time I did something competent at work, each time I was praised, I would add that experience, like a brick, to the fragile veneer of my professional self. It was a slow process. Back when I had just begun work, when I was asked to write my first article for an actual politician to go in an actual newspaper based on actual policy I had developed, I fell to pieces. I couldn't sleep. I could barely articulate when I was spoken to by the people I still considered as the *real* grown-ups. But over time I got more confident, each little triumph building on the last until I had enough ballast not to have to fake being an adult any more.

The turning point was around June 2007. Tony Blair was just leaving office, and Gordon Brown coming in. As usual with a change of PM, Downing Street was being hollowed out. All the political appointees (all the friends I had worked with over the past few years) were packing up their desks and leaving. Gordon's people were coming in. I was one of the few civil servants who were remaining, and had been put in charge of keeping people jolly during this strange handover. The bureaucrats lined the chequerboard lobby of No. 10 and clapped Tony out as he left for his new life. A swift rearrangement of the furniture and we were back in the same line, clapping Gordon in. Even though my world had shifted overnight, there was no room for reminiscing. Quite rightly, our new PM required us all to be on top form, straight away. Our allegiance to the new man had to be made clear. And so it was. Within seventy-two hours two car bombs were discovered in the West End, and there was an attempted terrorist attack on Glasgow Airport. We were in the middle of a manhunt, watching things play out live on Sky News, and because counter-terrorism was still within my ragbag of policy interests I was (notionally) in charge. Sleepless, anxious, and never feeling less like a grown-up I had to brief our new prime minister over those restless, strange first few days of his tenure. But by that point I had faked it enough times to know that I could make it in the grown-up world.

But my fragile professional edifice couldn't survive the bombardment of motherhood. When I eventually returned to the adult world of African politics after having the Knights, my boobs leaked both milk and self-assurance. I tried to hire a replacement bosslady, because I could not foresee a day when I would be able to do her job again. But somehow, over the months, I reconstructed myself as someone who was not just able, but allowed, to be in charge. Week after week of decisions, phone calls, meetings and memos slowly rebuilt the professional self that motherhood had torn down so violently. This time, it seemed built to last. My babymother-cum-CEO existence grew a very different sort of confidence in me. The archetypal working mother, I was more effective in one day than my colleagues could be in three, my ruthless efficiency born of the siren call the Knights emitted to pull me away from work. And oh, they made me fearless. What decision was too great when compared with the responsibility of being their mother? They crawled fast, and I had to keep up. I was impatient with people, restless for a pace at work that would match the relentless twenty-four-hour rhythm my babies had set for me. I was more than a little addicted to it all. In control, spinning plates, balancing a hundred different pieces of irreplaceable antique china. Never faltering for a moment. Craving the recognition and the praise that came with doing a good job. Loving the glowing red light on my BlackBerry just a little too much. I don't think I am alone in having felt all this. The professional self I had constructed was smart and well-dressed and had stimulating conversations with amazing people. People were impressed. Inhabiting her world was exhilarating.

Then I got punched in the face. The Nuisance finally declared itself, and within hours I had gone from having it all to losing it all. I recognised, the day after my diagnosis, that work as I knew it was over. Even if the bastard hadn't come back to finish me off, how could I go back to leaving my family for two weeks out of every four? How could I raise money for my charity when my family's financial future suddenly seemed so precarious? How could I write another word, except for my darling boys? So I stopped. I let go of it all – the big job, responsibility, ambition. Where once my armour was a series of smart dresses, fit for meeting presidents and philanthropic backers, now I lived in leggings, and only occasionally bothered to wear a bra. I watched those material embodiments of *Kate* fade away. I watched them fade with no regret, and – to my surprise – this time they didn't leave a void.

There was no void because that Kate – the one with hyper-robotic functionality and a kick-ass working wardrobe – well, she wouldn't have lasted long. Nuisance or no Nuisance, I suspect her time was limited. She would eventually have realised that she was not only entitled to some kind of intellectual hinterland behind the assembly line of life with twins and a big job, but that she *required* it to sustain everything else. My mum once said I was like Icarus – I flew too close to the sun. Cancer melted the wax that held my wings together, and I fell to earth. I know she didn't mean I brought terminal cancer on myself with my BlackBerry addiction. What she meant is that, like that of Icarus, my flight was not based on solid engineering. My wings were flimsy, and badly made. If it wasn't cancer, something else would have destroyed them. Or perhaps I would have willingly taken them off and contented myself with an existence on earth.

Now I've fallen, and it's not so bad down here. It seems that I am more than an oyster. I am the sum of all that I've done in the world – the people I've met, the lives I've touched, the choices I've made. The relentless forward motion is gone, but somehow my definition remains.

That is not to say that there is no sadness about losing the professional future I might have had. I am often torn between gratitude for this strangely fulfilling life I now have, and bitter resentment that I won't someday be running the UN. It would be surprising if this little tussle wasn't part of my mental architecture. Of course I miss being in the arena. Elections are torture; I long to be behind the black door again, privy to secrets, close to power. I worry that, tucked away in my little room, I will quietly become a bystander, one of the chorus, no longer connected to mankind as I was when the world was in my face every day. Oh, let my own predicament not slowly squeeze empathy out of my mental landscape, for then I truly will become a self-absorbed fiend. But still there is this unexpected sense of completeness. What a relief not to be clinging on to the edifice of my ambitious professional self as if *that* were going to save me from eradication. What a relief it is that I don't have to lean in to know who I am.

I wonder whether this unexpected sense of completeness stems from something else, something else which applies just as much to you lucky sods with decades ahead of you. I'm not doing what I was before, but I'm not doing nothing. I'm writing. The clickety-clack of my fingers on the keyboard is like the sound of rain on parched fields. Why did I ever stop doing this? If words are who I am, how did I let this become such a marginal part of my life? You know the answer, because I have described my neglected hinterland. It happens: work is, for most of us, what we do with our outer selves, the grown-up tip of the iceberg that we show the world, that which takes up our time and energy. But in all that aching and striving and achieving it is so easy to lose sight of the things which truly define us. These things try to break through, insistently, because they matter. I wonder now if part of my motivation for such frequent travel to Africa was the opportunities it offered me to swim in exotic places: the methane-filled waters of Lake Kivu, fearfully strong Atlantic seas at the inventively named River No. 2 Beach in Sierra Leone, dubious hotel swimming pools in Juba, Monrovia, Abuja, Conakry, Kigali, Blantyre and Jo'burg. Every year I spent longer than strictly necessary crafting our charity's annual report, a dry statutory requirement rather than a chance to show off my wordcraft – but a day locked in my attic writing *anything* was a treat.

Can it be that I was more sure of who I was at ten than at thirty? Is it possible that a small child can be closer to the holy grail of Maslovian self-actualisation than an adult? I think it is. The ten-year-old Kate knew what she liked. First, words. Second, swimming, and being outdoors. Third, playing. Behind these pursuits the insistent beat of an explorer's heart, a little girl who wanted to look the world in the eye, to know it, to be part of all the sadness and joy it contains. Now, none of my favoured childhood pursuits was going to turn me into *somebody*. But they were what gave me joy, and what does again now that I follow Mrs Dashwood from *Sense and Sensibility*'s advice to 'Know your own happiness.' Dying has freed me from convention and from ambition – now I work to live, to afford our next holiday or a bold new lipstick, to put money in the bank for my children's future. Dying has taken decades from me, but in the here and now it has given me back time to indulge in the things which sustain. I am coming full circle, my end is my beginning. Like Michael Mayne in his final months, I have become sure of my *cantus firmus*, the enduring melody of my life. I may prefer girl pop to the medieval Gregorian chants from which he derived the term, but I too can say:

This has been mine and mine alone ... there are certain truths and experiences that have seized and shaped me, and it is this firm ground that speaks to me of what is authentic, and to which I can return ... at every stage of this unpredictable human journey.

I follow my happiness, I return to my enduring melody.

I journey to other worlds, where I am a wild princess. Not the Disney kind: I am the sort who disguises herself as a boy in order to train as a knight, who then leads a retinue of brigands to conquer dragons and rescue her loyal prince. I have magic powers stronger than I can control at my young age. I can create potions to heal and to kill. I am a citizen of Narnia, of Brisingamen, of Middle Earth. My Knights and I journey to these places together. Now they lead me, now I lead them. I may be unable to use my bow and arrow to the devastating effect I once did, but I am a player nonetheless.

I feel my legs pushing through cold water, the sun on my face. I swim in English seas and remember all the other waters in which I have submerged myself. Alpine streams running over flat slabs of rock and forming cold pools to plunge into; tropical waterfalls reached after long walks through humid jungles; sea as clear as glass, soft sand and fish darting around coral reefs beneath my feet. I experience the joy of somersaulting through the water, doing handstands on the bottom of the pool. I can move in water like nowhere else. I am a naiad; in the water I don't care that I have so little hair and a podgy stomach chopped both on the horizontal and the vertical. I teach my children to swim and delight in their powerful limbs chugging through the water, my enthusiastic lessons a gift to the twins I have always called my little swimmers.

My synapses connect to pull words and memories out of grey matter. I take pleasure in stacking them together, in watching black type fill the page, where once it was my neat handwriting filling an exercise book with bad poetry and tales of weekends on the beach. Now I tap tap tap at the keyboard, taking my pleasure from plucking out the right word and slipping it next to another to explain this bizarre world I find myself in. I love to revisit what I write. Rearranging the words. Adding new ideas. Polishing a text is like polishing the stones my sister would collect; words whirr around my mind, becoming burnished and changed as I use them, like stones in the rock tumbler Jo cherished. I am salvaging something beautiful from the wreckage of our lives. Some days I feel as if I am reading my own mind only as the sentences form themselves. Words might slip, slide and perish – but so will I. And before then, they make a murky mess clear for me.

What would *your* ten-year-old self think if they could see you now? Would your *cantus firmus* ring out, or has it been deadened by the intervening years? Perhaps your former self would wonder why you no longer sing, or draw, or play the piano, or run, or make model aeroplanes. They might be confused by your interest in reading emails, and ask why you are not out in the rain making a wigwam instead. Do not dismiss their questions. We all put away childish things (I am not mourning the My Little Pony collection I once treasured). But amongst the discarded toys is what once made us happy, those passions and talents we indulged as children but which have since been put aside. So it turns out you aren't a chart-topping pop star, or a prize-winning artist. Making model aeroplanes doesn't pay the mortgage. You are better suited to a Saturday-morning run around the park than the Olympics. Who cares? We don't have to excel at something for it to matter, to make it part of who we are. Something doesn't have to be functional to be important.

I wonder if the same genius of humanity that lets us normalise so quickly through pain and torment also allows the water to close over our passions. One day we can't go a moment without writing poetry or playing the guitar; the next, those things are forgotten as if a distant dream. The quotidian routine, the rhythm of working life, anaesthetises so quickly. This helps. It is the reason I can function, but it is also the reason I spent so long forgetting all those things which give me joy. I wish I had remembered earlier that I had a right to a 'larger life' – an existence where my working self was connected to all the other creative, exploratory, curious selves I had long since discarded. In the meantime, I've missed out on a lot of front crawl and sword-fights.

Chase your happiness. Chase it down till you know who you are, because time past can also be time present, and those same things which once burnished your life can do so again.

9

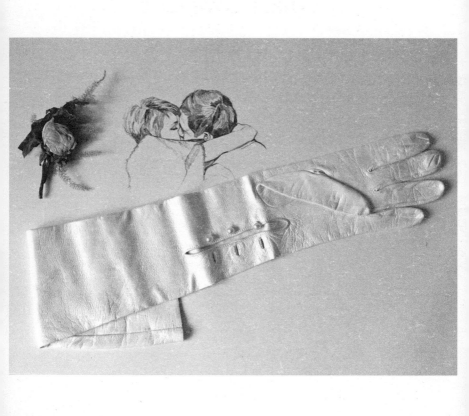

What's Love Got to Do With It?

To love at all is to be vulnerable. Love anything and your heart will be wrung and possibly broken. If you want to make sure of keeping it intact you must give it to no one, not even an animal. Wrap it carefully round with hobbies and little luxuries; avoid all entanglements. Lock it up safe in the casket or coffin of your selfishness. But in that casket, safe, dark, motionless, airless, it will change. It will not be broken; it will become unbreakable, impenetrable, irredeemable.

C.S. LEWIS, *THE FOUR LOVES*

Like most women my age, I have seen *Four Weddings and a Funeral* countless times. First, aged fifteen with Katie Milne Home at the sign-of-the-Nineties new multiplex in High Wycombe. Most memorably, escaping the monsoon rain in Mumbai, squashed into a small cinema near the India Gate. I always cry when John Hannah reads W.H. Auden's 'Funeral Blues'. When I was a grub I cried at the idea of love that strong (willing it to be Hugh Grant adoring me). Now I cry because Billy *is* my north, my south, my east and west. I cry because I imagine him at my funeral thinking that nothing now will ever come to any good. I cry when I think of him at home having put the boys to bed, alone on our sofa built for two, watching box sets without me. But I cry most when I think of Billy when he is sixty-five. He will still be handsome, his wide smile nestling amongst deep wrinkles, blue eyes twinkling away like a caricature of Irish good looks. For some reason I imagine him in an open-top sports car (strange, this, given it's neither his retirement dream nor mine). But I'm not in the passenger seat; someone else is. I am grieving for a future we won't have together. Nonetheless, I am the lucky one, because I never have to lose Billy. I get to face whatever I have to with him by my side. He doesn't have that luxury.

We met over a game of poker I was hosting. That sounds more risqué than it was. In reality my best woman had recently fallen in love with a young germanophile called Ian. Ian had a best friend (and much later a best man) called Billy. Billy and Ian were ace poker players; Jenny and I were not. Moreover, Jenny told me that Billy was absolutely not my type – handsome, yes, but facile and prone to tedious and drunken laddishness (you see, as I stalked the corridors of power with huge self-importance and limited self-awareness, what I thought I *really* needed was a mature older man). But then Billy and I met outside the bathroom of my rented flat in Clapham. One glance and I was deep into fantasy-land; he was the most beautiful man I had ever seen. And what's more, I had the in-a-movie feeling that we'd met before (perhaps *Once Upon a Dream*?). As far as I was concerned, this was 'IT'. The fairy tale I had always been told was out there: Cinderella and her prince, Hugh and Andie, Lizzie

Bennet and Mr Darcy all wrapped up into one romantic meeting outside the bog. After a little pursuit, Billy agreed to go out with me. We both made an effort for our early dates – he swotted up on the EU, and I grappled with ion mobility spectrometers. In a few months I was sitting on the 159 bus, moseying down the Kennington Road past the Imperial War Museum, musing about marriage. And though Billy was some way behind (only proposing to me after the Knights were born), two had become one, and we were tight.

I had been in love before, but not like this. You see, grubs only find other grubs to love. My relationships before Billy had been a series of unfortunate experiments. I was Pavlov's dog, and the smell of cheap aftershave was my buzzer, a siren call that drew me to grubs with nothing in their heads but football and fluff, disguised as handsome boys. It was a long time before I realised that relationships might offer a meeting of minds as well as bodies. The notion came upon me gradually, starting in Western Australia with a lovely chap to whom I read Bill Bryson on long car journeys, and with whom I made a special trip to see the stromatolites – the earliest ever form of life on earth – poking their stony little heads up in Shark Bay. And eventually, after much trial and even more error, there was Billy. Handsome like a movie star. A hinterland so large it would take me a lifetime to explore it. Generous, patient and challenging in equal measure. The very best sort of Austen hero: kind like Knightley, hot like Darcy.

We were feckless and irresponsible together for five blissful years. We worked hard in jobs that consumed us, unencumbered by demands on our hearts or pockets from little Knights, surrounded by friends doing the same. Billy commuted to Cambridge, I worked in Downing Street. Billy's company was in its infancy – he wooed American investors and built up his team making nanotech noses, clever minuscule widgets that can smell any chemical thrown at them. I sniffed the wind of politics and tried to work out what the leader of the opposition would throw at the prime minister every Wednesday. The first half of the week we spent apart, but on Wednesday evenings we would meet in a pub next to Trafalgar Square. It wasn't smart, but the beer was cheap. We drank too much, ate sushi in Soho and stumbled back to the flat we shared south of the river. At the weekends we got up late, wandered along the South Bank and went to the kind of messy parties thrown by feckless twenty-somethings. There I would watch Billy dance, something he only does with a beatific smile on his face and a pint in his hand. If I was lucky I would catch his eye and he would smile a smile only for me. While I am glad we had those days of courtship, the truth is I don't miss them. We were still feeling one another out, working out how much to pour into this new partnership. They were heady, exciting times. But my realisation on the 159 bus had made me excruciatingly vulnerable. I wanted this lovely man to be by my side forever, and wondered whether he felt the same.

Fortunately, something about me (perhaps my fine eyes, or my neatly turned ankles?) enraptured him sufficiently, and slowly our irresponsible romance became a responsible, grown-up love. I spent a week in Cambridge one hot June, eating scones in the shade at The Orchard and swimming in the lido on Jesus Green. This taste of life in a university town (albeit one stuck happily in the 1920s) convinced me to move out of London so that we could live together full-time. A year later, over a plate of raclette one evening in a down-at-heel ski resort in the Alps, we decided to have babies. Five years later, our love has lasted more than a decade. Billy has become my family, the person I turn to before anyone else, for everything.

Of course, there have been *Fuck you* moments, usually in the middle of the night as we pass each other in the corridor, each trying to quiet a howling baby, bitterly jealous of the amount of sleep we imagined the other to be getting. But over the years we have bent gently towards one another, Khalil Gibran's oak and cypress incarnate. Billy has learned, through the medium of the repetitive nag, that clothes do not spontaneously fly from floor to washing machine, and that there is no such thing as a bin angel. I discovered that although I was bosslady at work, Billy did not respond well to my challenging management style. The Knights glue us together. Having weathered the battlefield of the early years, we run a tight ship. We know how we fare when the vomit starts to fly, when the toys are thrown out of the pram, when the dog poo needs picking up.

Togetherness means intimacy, not homogeneity. Billy has abandoned his study of the finer points of EU comitology and development economics. Unsurprisingly, given my remedial physics, I never understood the inner workings of his little sniffing widgets, having got stuck at the bumper-sticker 'dime-sized detection' he used to pitch his invention to the Yanks. We have our own intellectual spaces. We have separate friends. Where Billy runs, I walk. He reluctantly puts on a pair of wellies for a muddy country outing with me; I reluctantly put up with his expensive technological fads invading the house.

The winds of heaven dance between us. Of course, the space where the wind blows could have grown into a chasm, as it can for any couple. The *Fuck you* moments could have overtaken the *I love you so much* moments (it is easy to accidentally cross the line from familiarity to incivility, and hard to row back from it once you have). Luck could have driven us apart – had I fulfilled my early promise and become forever a tetchy, dried-up husk of a worker bee, or had Eva Green moved to Cambridge in search of a job in a small nanotechnology start-up. My much-wanted third child (fictional little Josie) could have pushed our parenting abilities and our finances to their limit. So I try not to sentimentalise the future we won't have too much, because there is no guarantee that we would have had it. The long stretch of marriage I imagined for us takes work as well as luck, and I can only hope my better self would have carried on putting that work in.

What does illness do to a partnership like ours? We are still finding that out. Of course, our roles have changed. The woman who once leaned in now sits, and soon will only recline, and that makes for a different kind of home life and a different kind of Kate. Outwardly, we look less like equals. I appear the dependant, the one who gets driven around, cooked for and generally mollycoddled. I am allowed lie-ins and get taken on nice outings. In any and all clinical settings, if Billy isn't there I would prefer a light sedation to being alone. He is my talisman against the smells, the sounds, the vomit and the endless potential for bad news to arrive without warning. On the days we get my scan results, you can see us sitting side by side reading cheery Holocaust memoirs and occasionally squeezing one another's sweaty palms. But my dependence isn't the whole picture. While I'm here, I'm here. We are still two, not one. We argue and I grump around as I always have done. We negotiate on a daily basis what I can and can't do, because my worst days are when I can't manage the most basic of household tasks, and therefore feel like an utterly non-contributory member of the human race. Can I take the boys to school? Can I cook dinner? Can I unload the dishwasher and clean the floor? On my best days the negotiations are different: I'll take the boys swimming while you go for a run. I'll make waffles for breakfast. The list of what is and isn't possible goes up and down, but Billy understands that I need to contribute to the family to feel alive. So he never wraps me in cotton wool. I understand what he needs too, in the way you only really get when you sleep next to someone and understand their strange rhythms, little moods, odd foibles. I know when he needs to be out working up a manly sweat in his running shoes. I know when he needs to be in the pub drinking with his friends. And I know when he needs to be at home, next to me on the sofa, watching a box set with his head on my shoulder. So, while I am here, I am here, the comforter as well as the comforted, the parent and not only the parented, the cook, cleaner and Lego-builder-in-chief. Whatever it may look like to the outside world, the dependency between us passes two ways.

Of course, I wonder what will happen when things finally change and I lose my cherished independence. I know it will be Billy I want moistening my lips with water in my final hours. He won't need to tell me he loves me, he can just sit, safe in the knowledge he has made my already happy life golden. All I will want is for him to be there, quietly but permanently my north, my south, my east and west.

But I know, too, that even as I lie dying I will find room to be frustrated if he doesn't intuit my needs, to be irritated if he has the TV on too loud. Because normal breaks through, persistently, sometimes comically. Intimacy isn't made in perfection; it comes from the daily niggles as well as the power-ballad moments. I know this because through my weak and morphined haze after my liver operation Billy and I managed a terse little row. I was trying to explain that the drugs were making me hallucinate, and that I wanted to come off them. I demanded that the doctors come in to hear me out. But I couldn't actually speak, and anyway this inner dialogue was fighting for space with opiate-induced hallucinations of Las Vegas showgirls and African child soldiers who filled my hospital room. My ranting to Billy and to the doctor was an embarrassing torment for all concerned. But it was Billy I blamed, somehow furious with him for not reading my mind and lifting me out of this mental quagmire. So I know that even as he strokes my hair when I lie breathing my last, I shall be both beyond glad that he is there, and mildly irritated that he hasn't learned how to massage my feet. And I am certain that he will still allow himself to be annoyed by me, by my whimsical and incomprehensible demands, my dying-day nags. Love doesn't turn into sainthood just because it is suffused with suffering. It becomes more visceral – I simply cannot imagine facing this without him. But even in the most beautiful partnerships there is always space for our graceless natures to emerge, for the quotidian niggles true intimacy brings.

Because I love him, I project myself forward into a world where I am not there. I imagine Billy on his own of an evening, having dealt with endless bedtime questions from the Knights as to my whereabouts, and whether he is going to die and leave them too. Little hands clinging to him begging for another story, one final tuck-in. I wonder what that grief and loneliness will feel like, and how he will manage it. I wish more than anything that I could be there to help him through it, rather than be the cause of it all. I have tried to take myself to the place that he will find himself in by reading. C.S. Lewis's *A Grief Observed*, Joan Didion's *The Year of Magical Thinking*, and in my more desperate and less literary moments, online grief memoirs. I struggle. I struggle to imagine what it will be like. I have never lost anyone. I can glimpse for a moment what it might feel like, but I am unable (not unwilling) to take myself to the place he will inhabit. As Didion describes it:

> Grief turns out to be a place none of us know until we reach it ... Nor can we know ahead of the fact (and here lies the heart of the difference between grief as we imagine it and grief as it is) the unending absence that follows, the void, the very opposite of meaning.

Our bed is too big without him in it for one night, let alone a lifetime. I am exhausted by a weekend of solo parenting, let alone the next thirty years. At the end of a dinner with friends, I lean my head on his shoulder, never lonely in company because he is there. He shouldn't have to be without me.

Of course, being Billy, he doesn't show me much of his pain. He is by my side helping me live, not pre-visiting the grief he will feel in the future. Research tells me that the worst of it will be over after a few years. I have given my benediction to a future Mrs Boyle, though Billy won't even speak of it now. But in truth my feelings are more mixed. I want Billy to be happy and loved. I want someone to get the washing done, without the darks bleeding into the lights. If the two could combine in one washerwoman-cum-wife, ideally without my sparkling eyes and wit, perhaps I could look down on that content. But then I think about the imaginary convertible, driving off under East Anglian skies. Someone else with *my Billy*, seeing *my friends*. I imagine her in *my kitchen* telling the boys off for some teenage incursion. *My job*. I am haunted by this non-existent woman. I long for my best friend to scare her off, to try to hold my place in all their lives open indefinitely. There is no poetry, no great literature to help me with these rancorous feelings. I have to keep them in their place, squashed out of existence by a better, more generous me.

I find myself completely able to imagine the future Billy and I would have had. It is, somehow, far easier for me to project myself into it than it is for me to imagine the important moments of my children's lives – graduations, weddings, christenings.

Occasionally an image of a grown Isaac or Oscar crosses my mind, but I find it hard to conjure them up. Perhaps it is too painful. Perhaps I am giving them space to be who they will be. There is no such boundary when it comes to Billy. Despite the shadowy presence of another *her*, I still allow myself frequent daydreams of what might have been. I imagine a time when the boys are grown, happily, and we are no longer striving so hard for work, school, money. I imagine daytime trips to the cinema. I imagine Billy and me in America, silver-haired pensioners driving coast to coast (there's that convertible again), exploring enormous mountain ranges and wild beaches, boating in the sunshine on Central Park Lake just as we did when we were twenty-five. I imagine us buying a little white house next to the sea in Norfolk. There would be an open fire, and we would read contentedly alongside each other. I would finally learn to cook food he liked, stirring garlic and wine together as we talked and laughed about our children, our friends, our long lives together.

* * *

There are things I know about love, because of all this.

Good things come to those who wait. True Love's Kiss arrives only when you know yourself. Everyone who comes before is a frog, however good they smelled at the time.

Why not want love to last forever? I wanted someone to spend my whole life with. As Pelagia's wise old father advised in *Captain Corelli's Mandolin*, 'Love is not breathlessness, it is not excitement, it is not the promulgation of promises of eternal passion. That is just being "in love", which any of us can convince ourselves we are. Love itself is what is left over when being in love has burned away, and this is both an art and a fortunate accident.' How could you not want that? I am a newbie at marriage, so I understand if the more experienced among you regard what I have to say with a certain cynicism. But all I want is to be like Father Gregory Boyle's mum and dad in this passage from his memoir *Tattoos on the Heart: The Power of Boundless Compassion*:

I turn to see that my father has placed the flowery pillow over his face ... For the rest of the morning I catch him turning and savouring again the scent of the woman whose bed he has shared for nearly half a century.

When I consider what it is that makes me wish to all the pantheon of gods that I *had* half a century to spend with Billy, it is simple. I respect him. I respect his mind. It offers endless newness for me, because he is endlessly changing and therefore endlessly fascinating. Perhaps this is what people mean when they say you can fall in love with someone over and over again over the course of a marriage. I could so easily fall in love with forty-something Billy, fifty-something Billy, hey, eighty-something Billy. He is only going to get better and better.

A half-century together would only be possible with kindness; a dramatic, exciting hinterland on its own would only get me so far. I love Billy because he is tender and polite with me (even when I am a mean girl to him). We don't go to bed angry. He carries my heart in his, as tenderly as if it were his own.

Without love, I'd be gone already. There is no one else I want to face this with me. I need his clammy hand-squeezes as we wait to hear about the inexorable spread of this dreadful Nuisance. I need him to scoop me off the floor after chemotherapy. I need him as we speed into A&E as I vomit. I need him to be the reason I can keep going back for more and more treatment. I know there is something worse than dying, and that is dying alone. I wish I could share what Billy and I have with every poor sod I see sitting on their own in the hospital waiting room without their beloved next to them.

Finally, there is what I hope, because of all this. I hope that the old maxim that it is better to have loved and lost than never to have loved at all is really true. Let John Donne be right (he usually is): 'Filled with her love, may I rather be grown/Mad with much heart, than idiot with none.'

Sometimes I wonder if Billy wishes things were ordinary for him. An ordinary wife he didn't have to nurse. An ordinary marriage. Whole days without thinking about cancer or the latest clinical trials or pain relief. But then I put myself in his shoes. If I were the survivor, I would build our little family in an eternal homage to all that he was and could have been. I would wrap my grief up in their future. I would watch them grow, and see Billy every day in their faces. That wouldn't make it all right, but it would make it better. And I would read Viktor Frankl, and hold on to the image of Billy in my mind as a talisman, a reminder of my better self and all that matters in life.

My mind still clung to the image of my wife. A thought crossed my mind: I didn't even know if she were still alive. I knew only one thing – which I have learned well by now: Love goes very far beyond the physical person of the beloved. It finds its deepest meaning in his spiritual being, his inner self. Whether or not he is actually present, whether or not he is still alive at all, ceases somehow to be of importance.

I did not know whether my wife was alive, and I had no means of finding out (during all my prison life there was no outgoing or incoming mail); but at that moment it ceased to matter. There was no need for me to know; nothing could touch the strength of my love, my thoughts, and the image of my beloved. Had I known then that my wife was dead, I think that I would still have given myself, undisturbed by that knowledge, to the contemplation of her image, and that my mental conversation with her would have been just as vivid and just as satisfying. 'Set me like a seal upon thy heart, love is as strong as death.'

10

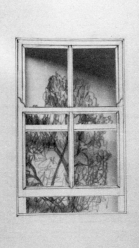

Sing, Everyone

I have loved the stars too fondly to
be fearful of the night

SARAH WILLIAMS, 'THE OLD ASTRONOMER

(TO HIS PUPIL)'

I have chosen the room where I would like to die. Not our bedroom, but the little study at the back of the house. Its large windows overlook the eucalyptus tree in the garden. It fits a single bed, a chair and a bookshelf. I figure that is about all I will need. Sleep, company, a nice view and something for people to read to me when I can no longer turn the pages myself. For a long time the room had a large aeroplane sticker on the wall with 'Oscar' written across it; but I have reclaimed it and filled it with clutter. It is a quiet, tranquil little void, not the noisy epicentre of our home. It can quickly be returned to its rightful function as a dumping ground for white-goods guarantees and school reports when I'm gone.

I am not afraid of ceasing to be. I am not preoccupied with what it means to be dead – there was a time when I was nothing, and there will be a time when I am nothing again. Our little lives are rounded with a sleep: first the sleep of a newborn, then the sleep of the dying. I am not scared of that drowsiness, nor am I consumed by thinking about what it will be like. As someone said to me, your day isn't defined by the moments before you drift off. It is the part when you are awake that counts.

I say this, of course, from a comfortable sofa in Cambridge. There is still time for me to lose it, to die the opposite of a dignified death (whatever that is). I reserve the right to fall apart at a later date. I am not afraid of ceasing, but I am afraid of the weeks of twilight, pain and decline that precede it. What if I unravel as my body starts to deteriorate? Will the cancer spread to my brain? If the tumours spread to my grey matter I'm done for, emotionally, because that will finally rob me of the only thing I thought it couldn't – my brain, myself, my me. I sometimes wonder if I can handle dying only if I am well. I realise this sounds like an insane oxymoron, but the point is that physical strength and absence of pain provide mental and emotional resilience. I know from enduring years of treatment that when I am in pain I grow further from myself, mentally. You know what it feels like when you have a throbbing hang-over; the world seems a crueller and more difficult place when it's hard to lift your head from the pillow.

So, this book needs to finish at the end. With death. With struggle between the me that has been *All right so far*, even through all this crap, and the spectre of a me who finally falls apart. I know which ending I prefer, so I will write it, and will it to be the truth. I will myself to die a classy death, like my literary role-model, Charity Lang – 'She will burn bright till she goes out; she will go on standing on tip toe till she falls.'

*   *   *

I will start with the good news. There is an unutterably brilliant secret which has made all of this horror bearable, which has made things All Right so far. I have kept it to the end of the book, though I am sure you have worked it out long ago. To paraphrase the much-quoted words of a good, solid Victorian poet, you are the captain of your soul. What happens to you, uncontrollable or otherwise, isn't the important thing. What matters is simply how you *are* with it. And you can always, always, choose that. Knowing this provides meaning and purpose even amidst the greatest pain and sadness. Back to Viktor Frankl:

> The way in which a man accepts his fate and all the suffering it entails, the way in which he takes up his cross, gives him ample opportunity – even under the most difficult circumstances – to add a deeper meaning to his life. It may remain brave, dignified and unselfish. Or in the bitter fight for self-preservation he may forget his human dignity and become no more than an animal. Here lies the chance for a man to either make use of or to forgo the opportunities of attaining the moral values

that a difficult situation may afford him. And this decides whether he is worthy of his sufferings or not ... Such men are not only in concentration camps. Everywhere man is confronted with fate, with the chance of achieving something through his own suffering.

While I don't have a choice about cancer, or dying, I do have a choice. I have a choice about how I live with it and how I die. I've had a great life. I still have a great life. What's the point in spending the last chapter of it being sad? You might expect to find me depleted, fretful, full of grief. You won't. I am growing fat on the marrow of life (I grant you, the steroids are also helping me stay rotund). I assert that wonder and joy are more powerful than the sadness of a truncated life. I made this choice early on, returning to wry Jonathan Swift, who tells us to 'live all the days of our life', and to Billy's beloved Montaigne:

The utility of living consists not in the length of days, but in the use of time; a man may have lived long, and yet lived but a little. Make use of time while it is present with you. It depends upon your will, and not upon the number of days, to have a sufficient length of life.

When I first found myself identifying with this kind of sentiment, I was horrified at my effortless slide into cancer cliché. Self-aggrandisement told me my experience of living for the moment was unique, and needed to be shared, even as I feared becoming just another 'Livestrong' story. But of course other people have trodden this path, and my strangely joyful experience of suffering is actually a common one. All I can do is explain it in a way which is as far from the saccharine cancer bumper-stickers and sponsored-walk T-shirts as I can manage.

Obviously, to do this I have to resort to other people's words. Our joys are our sorrows unmasked, and in our sorrow we have found great joy. What is *your* daily bread is *my* greatest pleasure. I sit at the kitchen table with my boys as they draw scenes of Viking battles and I feel settled. I watch as they run into ice-cold seas and their crazy exuberance mirrors what is going on, albeit more quietly, inside my heart. I have my afternoon snooze on their bunk bed and wake to the sounds of them crashing through the door as they return from school, and I am perfectly content to be where I am right in that perfect little moment. As a family we make and execute rash plans: a huge wedding in the middle of my most gruelling chemotherapy; climbing mountains (well, one small one); gathering oldest and dearest friends together for wild parties; the purchase of a puppy in place of the baby we won't now have. And through all of this we have the little moments of wonder which let the light in. Pink tulips under a crowd of silver birches. Ely Cathedral rising from the flatlands. Frogs spawning in the pond at Mum and Dad's. Dancing to Bruce Springsteen in the kitchen. It reminds me of the Frank O'Hara poem so often read at weddings; 'Having a Coke with you/is even more fun than going to San Sebastian, Irún, Hendaye, Biarritz, Bayonne'. Drinking the Coke together is all I really need. The rest is garnish.

More of someone else's words:

I moved my chair into sun
I sat in the sun
the way hunger is moved when called fasting.

I sent this poem by Jane Hirshfield to all our beloveds after the news that my cancer had returned. I like to think it tapped into today's zeitgeisty fad, the fast diet, through which half our social circle has lost their burgeoning middle-aged spread. If they can transmute ravenous hunger and a compelling desire for afternoon biscuits into something which they have chosen to do, then they can understand why, contrary to their expectations, life is good for us. We aren't existing in some state of suspended animation as I slip away; we are living, just as they are. We don't require kid gloves. We want to go with them on holiday. We want to play after school. Everything has changed and yet nothing has changed. In other words, the petty frustrations and stupid ambitions and general rushing around have melted away, but the good stuff remains.

And it's better than ever. And so here you have the unexpected, glorious secret about dying. When you know it is going to happen, you can choose to make the final chapter of the story the very best one of all.

I am trying not to leave you with the impression that I am some kind of saint who translates sorrow into bliss through the sheer power of her inner glow. It is true that some people are using the news of my early demise as a chance to beatify me. I am not resisting this very hard, because I am vain, and who would tire of letters that say they are brave and inspirational? But I'm afraid the beatified Kate is just a cipher, a way for people to feel OK about my looming grave without really confronting the truth of our family's experience. Really, sainthood would be dull, as much an abdication of my real self as slipping away quietly like Beth from *Little Women*. I am scared of the future, that the joy and wonder will finally evaporate when things get worse. I am a grumpy pain on a Sunday evening. I nag poor Billy about keeping the car clean. I think and often say terrible things about my children, and though I count the days I get to spend with them, still I am relieved when the summer holidays are over. I can still be a mean girl. I lie and say I'm not well enough to see people just because I can't be bothered. I am short with people in call centres and mobile-phone shops, and at tedious social functions (I like to think I have a good excuse, but really I'm just rude). While I am very much living all the days of my life, that doesn't mean I am or need to be happy every day. Living is about feeling angry, irritable and sad too. I enjoy my quiet, surly, mean-spirited days as much as the days when I am full of joy and wonder. They remind me that I still have red blood pumping through my veins.

I struggle with time, because I don't know how long this glorious final chapter will be. The seasons have a different meaning now. Inside the grey domes of the MRI or CT machines, hospitals show 'uplifting' pictures to help patients pass the time during the interminable scans. In January they showed a spread of magnolia flowers. Pinned down on my back, machines whirring, my body sliced and diced by a million tiny rays, I cried and cried at the thought that I might not see the real magnolias come out. When they arrived I caressed their waxy petals like talismans. Spring passed by on hyper-speed. Red tulips destroyed by vigorous games of football. The pink clematis that every year marks the boys' birthday gone in a flash. Purple alliums, followed by fat white peonies shedding their petals too fast. Every day I want to press Pause and soak in each moment, but the next comes on too fast, and I am dazzled by it all. I want to press Pause not just because I am petrified that I won't experience each of these moments again (though that I am), but because I want to suck the marrow out of them, to make myself experience the waxy petals as intensely as if they were my own flesh. I wish I didn't feel the insistent *whoosh* of Time's winged chariot behind me, but I do, I do. And it makes me panic. Not about dying, or not *purely* about dying. More that I haven't *appreciated* the tulips, the clematis, the alliums, the peonies, the honeysuckle, enough. Soon they will be over, and what if I didn't notice them properly while I had the chance?

This is the problem with my least favourite cancer cliché, the bucket list. In what universe is it OK to say that I have climbed Slieve Donard, or canoed down the Aveyron gorge, or blubbed through my kids' nativity play for the last time? I'm not in denial – in my heart of hearts I know that I've probably seen my last Balearic sunset and eaten my last Parisian éclair. But acknowledging the lastness of an experience elevates it to an unbearable level of meaning. You could spend the entire time you were sky-diving over the Grand Canyon clouded by a sense of sadness and impending doom, petrified that you are somehow not 'in the moment' enough, or not enjoying yourself sufficiently. I fell into this trap early on. When I left hospital after my diagnosis and first operation, back in October 2012, I imagined I'd be bedridden forever. I thought my swimming days were done, though of course they weren't. Likewise, later on, I was terrified the first time I had to ask someone else to pick the kids up from school in my place. I assumed that was the beginning of the end, that they would never see my cheery face in the playground again. But I perked up a few weeks later. Everything is just a phase, when it comes down to it, whether a good one or a bad one. Life is continual flux. Things go up and down. So there is a perversely optimistic logic to my refusal to acknowledge lastness. Anyway, who knows? There might still be time to squeeze in one more éclair.

Writing this book is, of course, my most powerful rebuke to the insistent hoof-beat of the horse and his accursed driver, Time, so smug and domineering in his winged chariot. The urge to create something permanent when your own impermanence is revealed is as old as time. Like Keats, I imagine dying before 'high-piled books, in charact'ry/Hold like rich garners the full-ripen'd grain'. I suspect that things were slightly more tricky for him, as an unpublished, ambitious twenty-something man with something *truly* great to say, than they are for me. Frankly, I feel lucky that I have this opportunity to spill out my half-ripen'd grain to you. There is something biological about it. I won't have more children. I will leave the children I have motherless. But though I am breaking the laws of nature, destroying the perfect two-by-two unit of family with my death, still I can create *something*. Even as I'm on the way out, something new is being spawned. I die, but in doing so I leave myself in words on a page, waiting to be brought alive by the two readers I care most about in the world.

I couldn't not write this book. But the writing of it is problematic in itself. In darker moments I catch myself wondering who I am really writing for. Is this an essentially selfish endeavour? Am I replacing my old striving for academic or professional success with a new sort of striving – this time for immortality? Should I really be writing, instead of picking my children up from school? I wonder if they would cherish the memory of more time with me over these words. Perhaps I am no better than medieval patriarchs going round whoring and impregnating so that their bloodline would live on forever. There are evenings when my patience is strained at story time, when I snap at Billy because I have spent my day writing when I should have been sleeping. At these moments I compare myself, unfavourably, to the less selfish cancer patients I have read about in my grim perusal of deathbed memoirs. One had this quote perpetually by her side:

This is of great importance, to watch carefully –
now I am so weak – not to over fatigue myself,
because then I cannot contribute to the pleasure
of others; and a placid face and a gentle tone will
make my family more happy than anything else I
can do for them.*

I read this and I am curdled with self-loathing. My
face is not placid, my tone not gentle. I am a
monstrous, selfish mother and wife. But the truth is,
I always have been. I place my own needs high in the
scale of things, and I'm not afraid to look after
myself. I explain to myself that I was a better mother
because I worked, because I had a public as well as a
private life. Therefore I will be better at dying if that
same part of me stays alive for as long as she can.

Time rushes on. Like John Donne's lovers in 'The
Anniversary', we can't make the sun stand still, but

---

* By Elizabeth T. King, quoted in Will Schwalbe's *The End of
Your Life Book Club*.

we make it run for its life as we squeeze every last bit of joy from my truncated existence. We are getting good at predicting when it will shine, and when it does we sit in it, basking in the warmth it creates (you see, even my poetic metaphors overrun themselves with exuberance).

But I suspect this is only possible because of something else I have done. It should be abundantly clear by now that I am a chronic control freak. I think I have been able to get on with living because I have looked the end in the eye. When I was planning my wedding I embroiled myself in the detail of things. 'Wedmin', it is called in today's slang. Now I embroil myself in deathmin. I'm trying to set in place all that I can, because it's *my job* (even in death I find it hard to lose control). I hate the thought of leaving things undone. I hate the idea of leaving messy, crappy, administrative loose ends for Billy to deal with when all I want him to do is wrap the boys in soft towels after their bath and tuck them into bed with a kiss. This is why I have chosen the room I want to die in; this is why I have sought out palliative care experts to understand what my final weeks might be like; this is why I have completed an advance directive explaining that I'd rather not be given morphine if it gives me visions of genocide again. I have visited the hospice and met the nurses there who will care for me. I have sorted out my finances, and engaged in long email discussions with my employers about precisely how long I have to live to be eligible for the payout that will halve our mortgage. I have asked my best woman to read Siegfried Sassoon's 'Everyone Sang' at my funeral, and chosen the (various) places my ashes will rest. I have stopped short of deciding what outfit I should be cremated in and finding a venue for my memorial service, but only just. I suppose I should leave people with something to keep them busy.

My poor boys are the subject of the worst control-freak tendencies. Not only am I writing this book – a wordy *me me me* treasure map to follow when they want to – I am, according to my mum, doing some serious 'advance mothering'. As well as my reverse-nesting, as well as writing The Family Manual, I have begun to record myself reading bedtime stories so that the Roald Dahl back catalogue will be available in my dulcet tones. There will be a bookshelf in their room replete with all the books I would have encouraged (bribed, cajoled, ordered) my children to read. Willard Price (in lieu of *Ballet Shoes*) for now. Philip Pullman's *His Dark Materials* forever. *The Catcher in the Rye* for their teenage years. Milton. Peter Hennessy's history of British prime ministers. *The Oxford Book of Verse*. So many more, ordered by age, ordered by theme. At some point there will be money for the boys to travel the world, accompanied by those who know and love me. I want them to be global citizens, not little Englanders; to sit astride the world like a colossus. And there are the cardboard boxes stuffed with things which are special to us, things which I hope will jog a memory in them when they are grown. The books tell you to make these boxes, to spray your perfume over them. I'm not sure if the stones I have gathered from our holidays on East Anglian beaches will mean much to the boys in twenty years, but they feel smooth and cold in my hand as I pack the boxes up, and perhaps that is enough.

My counsellor told me that in more than ten years at the local hospice she had never met someone who faced death as straightforwardly as me. I am not at all sure she meant this as a compliment. She and others might feel more comfortable if there were more tears and fewer lists. I had a memorable visit to my GP to discuss 'end of life care', and some poor trainee medics were sent in to interview me ('What brings you to the surgery today?' 'I've got terminal cancer and I want to discuss palliative pain relief.' Awkward silence follows as they shuffle their notes). They were about eighteen, and left the room blind-sided and probably reconsidering their career choices.

It is easy to interpret my pragmatism as coolness, self-defence, hiding from pain in practicalities. There is some truth there. These fragments I have shored against my ruins, and all that. But I'm no idiot. I realise that all of this organisation is just papering over the gaping cracks that my absence will leave. I can't fix the future any more than I can fix the now; and anyway, my plans will only take the family so far – about a year Afterwards, I predict, then the lists will become obsolete and my family will have to fend for themselves. Really, I should just trust that they can do that without me. But despite all these labours,

I still spend more time than I should wondering whether, in the endless Afterwards, there will always be a pile of dirty socks under the sofa.

Afterwards is, for me, the state my family will exist in. It is the world that will go on without me. I am not much given to wondering what Afterwards will be like for Kate herself. We are clear that Billy will tell the boys that I am in heaven; for little minds schooled in Catholicism that is, for now, the right answer. In any event, where I end up is not something which troubles me very much. I feel simultaneously certain that my atoms will dissolve and that I will simply cease to exist – just as I didn't exist before July 1978 – and at the same time, that somehow I will be around, part of the fabric of the world I inhabited. More from my literary doppelgänger, Charity Lang: 'We'll stay right here where we loved it when we were alive. People will drink us with their morning milk and pour us as maple syrup over their breakfast pancakes.' Perhaps, rather than in the morning waffles I will hover around in the wind, watching all the good times while being completely shielded from any sadness my beloveds might ever experience, just as Ewan MacColl describes in his lovely song 'Joy of Living':

Take me to some high place of heather, rock and
    ling
Scatter my dust and ashes, feed me to the wind
So that I will be part of all you see, the air you are
    breathing
I'll be part of the curlew's cry and the soaring
    hawk,
The blue milkwort and the sundew hung with
    diamonds
I'll be riding the gentle wind that blows through
    your hair
Reminding you how we shared in the joy of
    living.

I feel certain about this because there are dead people who continue to inhabit my life. Three people in particular. They died aged fifteen, nineteen and twenty-five – hit by a car, of pneumonia, and by a roadside bomb in Iraq respectively. I wasn't particularly close to any of them, not in the grand scheme of things. If they were alive, I can't say we'd still be in touch now. But as it is, they are all gone, long before their time was up. And I think of them all the time. I always have. I can picture their faces better than I can some of my oldest friends. I remember the things they loved, the conversations we had. My nineteen-year-old friend and I sat on the roof of the school we taught at in Rajasthan, drinking cold beers. He told me about his older sister, affection I suspect he never showed her peeping out in the way he described their childhood together. I imagine him running butt naked into the sea in Goa, or on the back of a motorbike in Udaipur, perpetually the teenage explorer with soulful brown eyes, doing the things he loved. He is still here with me, present in my morning milk and maple syrup. And if he is here with me, someone I only knew for a brief moment in time, what does that mean for me and my beloveds? I suspect that for a long time my little family will no longer be four people, but they won't be just three either.

When it comes to the afterlife, I think my intellectual laziness is having a field day, and I'm very grateful for it. Contradictions in my thinking don't trouble me at all. Having said that, I do ask most of my visitors, especially the godly ones, what *they* think about the afterlife. I am fascinated by the faith people have that there is something concrete there to look forward to. But my fascination covers my lack of comprehension; I struggle with those who tell me that they really, truly believe in a heaven. I struggle not because of the leap of faith it requires, but because I fail to see how anything *anywhere* else could be better than what we have right here, right now. Why would I want to be surrounded by celestial angels? Obviously it would be quite fun to hang out with Elizabeth I and Sylvia Plath – for a day – but then I'd just start wondering what was going on in the real world. And missing the smell of wet grass, and newly unfurling leaves, and of the boys' skin when they climb into bed with me in the morning. Frankly, I prefer my intellectually incoherent view of nothingness-with-benefits. More than that, I prefer to spend my time thinking about how we build the republic of heaven here on earth, which seems so much more fruitful.

I shall end this by reminding you to put your superhero glasses on, to pay attention to the wonder all around you. To get your dodgy bottoms checked out. To always, *always* eat from your very best crockery, because where can we live but days? To be as grateful as I am that you love, and are beloved.

And did you get what
you wanted from this life, even so?
I did.
And what did you want?
To call myself beloved, to feel myself
beloved on the earth.

RAYMOND CARVER, 'LATE FRAGMENT'

Acknowledgements

I need to try to restrict this to thanking people who have made this book happen, rather than everyone who has ever helped us (because otherwise this would be the Oscars acceptance speech of cancer memoirs). So, I would like to thank my agent Judith Murray and my editor Arabella Pike for taking a punt on me, believing that this wouldn't be just another cancer memoir, and for sharing my enthusiasm for books, shoes and make-up all the way through my many redrafts. Huge appreciation to all those who have read and commented on this book, especially my mum, Paul and Cruffy (who all deserve to be in print much more than I do). My talented friends Nadia and Becs provided the photos and illustrations which bring some of my memories alive, and Sarah created the wonderful plate of my spiral drawing. Countless others contributed to this book, whether they know it or not. So, to all the inspirational people in the inner, middle and outer reaches of the spiral: thank you for squeezing my hand, feeding my mind and sharing your stories with me, and thank you for not complaining when I shared them with the world in this book.

Heartfelt thank-yous need to be said to the many wonderful nurses and medics who have treated me with such kindness, prolonged my life so I could write this, and told me bad news with as much grace as Raymond Carver's doctor.

And of course, thank you to Billy and the Knights for permitting me to write about our family in such an intimate way. It has helped me more than I can express, and I hope that it will help you too, in the great big Afterwards.

Bibliography

There could be a whole additional volume on the books which have shaped me. But here's my shortlist – many of those I've used in this book, and some of the other special ones which influenced me but didn't quite make it in. I've organised them according to when I first read them, so you can pick up what might be relevant to you at a similar point in your life.

With my back to the radiator
C.S. Lewis, *The Narnia Chronicles* (especially *The Horse and His Boy* and *The Dawn Treader*)

J.R.R. Tolkien, *The Hobbit* and *The Lord of the Rings*

Pat O'Shea, *The Hounds of the Morrigan*

Noel Langley, *The Land of Green Ginger*
Roald Dahl, *Matilda* and *The Witches*
All of Agatha Christie
Alison Uttley, *A Traveller in Time*
Louisa May Alcott, *Little Women*
Noel Streatfeild, *Ballet Shoes* and *The Painted Garden*
Lorna Hill, the *Sadler's Wells* series
Philip Pullman, *His Dark Materials* trilogy
Tamora Pierce, the *Song of the Lioness* quartet

The grub years
Margaret Mitchell, *Gone With the Wind*
Lynne Reid Banks, *The L-Shaped Room*
Sylvia Plath, *The Bell Jar* and *Selected Poems*
J.D. Salinger, *The Catcher in the Rye*
Toni Morrison, *Beloved*
William Shakespeare, *Hamlet*
Dodie Smith, *I Capture the Castle*
Nancy Mitford, *The Pursuit of Love*
Harper Lee, *To Kill a Mockingbird*
Arthur Miller, *The Crucible*

Emerging from the cocoon

William Dalrymple, *In Xanadu* and *City of Djinns*

Helen Fielding, *Bridget Jones's Diary*

John Milton, *Paradise Lost* and *Areopagitica*

William Langland, *Piers Plowman*

John Donne, *Collected Poems*

William Blake, *Collected Poems*

(Finally) William Shakespeare, *Complete Works*

Jane Austen, *Pride and Prejudice* and *Persuasion*

The woman in the arena

Rachel Cusk, *A Life's Work*

Ryszard Kapuściński, *The Shadow of the Sun*

Dennis Kavanagh and Anthony Seldon, *The Powers Behind the Prime Minister*

Peter Hennessy, *The Prime Minister: The Office and its Holders Since 1945*

Barack Obama, *Dreams From My Father*

John Keay, *Sowing the Wind: The Seeds of Conflict in the Middle East*

Philip Gourevitch, *We Wish to Inform You that Tomorrow We Will be Killed With Our Families*

Thomas Hobbes, *Leviathan*

Adam Smith, *The Wealth of Nations*

David Smith, *Free Lunch: Easily Digestible Economics*

Paul Collier, *The Bottom Billion: Why the Poorest Countries are Failing and What Can be Done About It*

Chris Mullin, *A View From the Foothills*

Philip Gould, *The Unfinished Revolution: How the Modernisers Saved the Labour Party*

Michael Mayne, *This Sunrise of Wonder: A Quest for God in Art and Nature*

End of life book club

Viktor Frankl, *Man's Search for Meaning*

T.S. Eliot, *Collected Works*

Emily Dickinson, *Collected Works*

Sarah Bakewell, *How to Live: A Life of Montaigne in One Question and Twenty Attempts at an Answer*

Michael Mayne, *The Enduring Melody*

Philip Gould, *When I Die: Lessons From the Death Zone*

John Diamond, *C: Because Cowards Get Cancer Too*

Ruth Picardie, *Before I Say Goodbye*

Bibliography

Will Schwalbe, *The End of Your Life Book Club*

Joan Didion, *The Year of Magical Thinking*

Father Gregory Boyle, *Tattoos on the Heart: The Power of Boundless Compassion*

Wallace Stegner, *Crossing to Safety*

Raymond Carver, *Complete Works*

Emily Rapp, *The Still Point of the Turning World: A Mother's Story*

Siddhartha Mukherjee, *The Emperor of All Maladies: A Biography of Cancer*

Postscript

Kate died at home in the room she'd chosen and prepared on 25 December 2014 at 6.29 a.m. Ten minutes before Oscar and Isaac asked 'Is it morning?' – so just long enough for Billy to hold her hand and say goodbye before stocking-opening, which of course cannot be delayed.

She had time to see and talk to the people who mattered to her most, to wrap and label the presents for the stockings, to give any number of directions about what should go where. She had time, too, to see the first copies of this book and to write inscriptions in them for her family.

Her last two weeks were characterised by the same qualities that marked her life. There was care for others: Were we all OK? Would we be OK? How could she make it OK for us? There was a decision not to complain. And there was a fierce need to control and order ('What's the plan? But what is the plan?'). Rather than sinking gently into the arms of diamorphine – she thoroughly disliked its parallel bonkers world, although the dreams this time were not the scary ones she had feared – for as long as she could, she sought to stay connected, and sane.

Her friends sent memories, films, photographs and poems. One day the postman brought a precise, delicate and surreal black-and-white picture on glass, by the artist who created Kate's spiral of support on a painted plate. Titled 'A Blissful Day', the picture shows Kate and the boys running hand in hand, Isaac flying above in superhero mode, Billy in a deckchair in the sun, King's College chapel, an elephant, two Knights in the distance, Aslan. All things that those who read this book will know as Kate.

There were tributes also from people who knew her public face, the woman in the arena, changing the world one paperclip at a time. One said, 'Kate was an inspiration when she was with us. She will

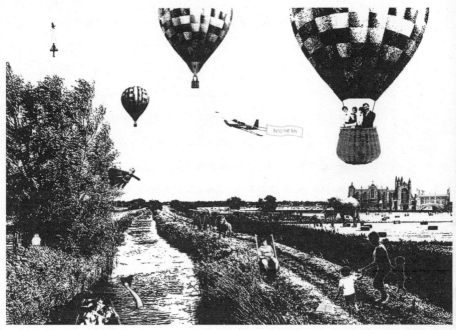

(courtesy of Sarah Curley)

remain an inspiration now and for the future. She was a life changer and a life giver.' We recognise that Kate, too.

And there was something else the Knights will like one day, when they have read this book. It was sent to Kate by a fellow author. Charlotte Brontë, reading her mother's letters in 1850 (her mother had died in 1821), wrote:

A few days since, a little incident happened which curiously touched me. Papa put into my hands a little packet of letters and papers, telling me that they were Mamma's, and that I might read them. I did read them, in a frame of mind I cannot describe. The papers were yellow with time, all having been written before I was born. It was strange now to peruse, for the first time, the records of a mind whence my own sprang; and most strange, and at once sad and sweet, to find that mind of a truly fine, pure, and elevated order. They were written to Papa before they were married. There is a rectitude, a refinement, a constancy, a modesty, a sense, a gentleness about them indescribable. I wish she had lived, and that I had known her.

We are all so glad to have known her.

Jean Gross, Kate's mother
31 December 2014